CHINESE MEDICINE

IN THE SAME SERIES:

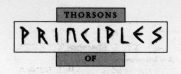

CHINESE MEDICINE

ANGELA HICKS

Thorsons
An Imprint of HarperCollins*Publishers*

An imprint of HarperCollins*Publishers*
77–85 Fulham Palace Road,
Hammersmith, London W6 8JB
1160 Battery Street,
San Francisco, California 94111–1213

Published by Thorsons 1996

10 9 8 7 6 5 4 3 2 1

© Angela Hicks 1996

Angela Hicks asserts the moral right to
be identified as the author of this work

A catalogue record for this book
is available from the British Library

ISBN 0 7225 3215 6

Printed in Great Britain by
Caledonian International Book Manufacturing Ltd, Glasgow

TO MY MOTHER AND FATHER

CONTENTS

AUTHOR'S NOTE

This book is written as an informative guide to Chinese medicine and is not meant as a self-help book for treatment.

After much consideration I have written this book in the feminine pronoun throughout. This is not meant as any slight to the 50 per cent of the population that are male. It is merely that I have had to make a choice and the English language does not yet provide a neutral pronoun that I could use. I have also capitalized all Chinese medicine terminology in order to differentiate them from standard English terms.

ACKNOWLEDGEMENTS

My thanks to all of the people who have helped me to write this book.

First, thank you to all of my patients who talked with me about their experiences of acupuncture. Thanks also to the patients of Tony Brawn and Caroline Root who allowed me to interview them about their experiences of taking herbs, patients of Sarah Pritchard who talked about receiving tui na and patients of Jill Glover and Leslie Jenkins who discussed changes in their diet. Thanks as well to all of those people who informed me of their experiences of practising qigong or who filled in questionnaires about it. The names of all patients have been changed to protect confidentiality.

Secondly, thanks to those practitioners who helped me with essential information that I have used in this book, especially Robert Cran and Sarah Pritchard who talked about tui na. Thanks also to my qigong teacher Dr Shen Hongxun who teaches Buqi healing, Taijiwuxigong, Taiji 37 and Wuxi meditation. He allowed me to use much of his theory including 'the three places on the spine to keep good posture', 'three methods for strengthening the tan tien', 'some useful eye exercises', as well as the three qigong exercises in this book, 'basic standing

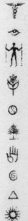

x posture', 'circling qi in the tan tien' and 'dragon swimming exercise'.

Finally, thanks to all those who have helped me by reading through parts of this book, most notably Judith Clark for painstakingly reading each new chapter, Ilana Pearlman for her many useful comments, Anna Barrie for teaching me to edit and Peter Mole who helped me with the 'big picture' and gave me so much helpful advice.

Many people have helped me to deepen my appreciation of Chinese medicine. J. R. Worsley trained me to understand the underlying essence of a patient. Vivienne Brown, Peter Deadman, Giovanni Maciocia and Julian Scott taught me about the basics of Chinese Medicine as it is used in China. I am very grateful to them for opening new doors in my understanding. I'm also grateful to Rose Gladden the healer who, while she was alive, was a major influence on my awareness of wholistic treatment and healing the spirit.

Many thanks and love to John, my husband, who as always supported and encouraged me when I was writing this book.

INTRODUCTION

I first became interested in Chinese medicine through a friend. I had known her for a long time but hadn't seen her for over a year. We arranged to meet in a restaurant and I was late. I walked in, looked around, and realized that she hadn't arrived yet either. There was only a romantic couple, a middle-aged businessman and a bright-looking young woman.

The young woman spoke to me, 'Hello Angela, have you gone blind? You looked straight at me then ignored me.' It was my friend. I hadn't recognized her because she looked so different. The story emerged as we chatted. She was having acupuncture treatment.

'I used to feel so low in energy all the time. The world looked very grey and it was an effort to get up in the morning. I had terrible headaches and permanent backache. I couldn't imagine life being any different and I used to feel really sorry for myself.

'After only five treatments I was feeling very different. I noticed I had a spring in my step and I felt lighter. I even began to look forward to work. That was really something! After some more treatment my body stopped aching and I began to feel much younger. It was almost as if a weight had slipped off me and I felt more "myself" than I had for years.'

She was very excited by what she was telling me. I was so

impressed that it wasn't long before I had decided that I wanted to change my career and learn acupuncture. I have now been practising for 20 years and have never looked back.

Chinese medicine was relatively unknown at the time and acupuncture was the main treatment available. Reference to 'acupuncture' let alone 'Chinese medicine' two decades ago was often met with a blank look or possibly an expression of puzzlement. Many doctors at that time showed hostility at their very mention.

Now 'acupuncture' is a familiar word to most people and many understand it to be a form of medical treatment where needles are used to cure illness. Chinese herbs are also well known to much of the population and qigong and tui na are fast catching up from behind. All of them are available in the West. Their rise in popularity has been happening quietly yet rapidly.

Many doctors now actively encourage their patients to have acupuncture or another form of Chinese medicine. Some Chinese medicine practitioners are being asked to work in clinics alongside their General Practitioners.

So why has the popularity of acupuncture and the other Chinese medicines spread so quickly? There are four main reasons:

1 The major reason is Chinese medicine itself. It works! People have voted with their feet. Word of mouth is perhaps the best advertisement and patients have recommended it because treatment is often successful. We might ask ourselves, 'Would it have survived for over 2,000 years if it wasn't effective?'

2 People are now much more conscious of the importance of good health. Twenty years ago the diagnosis and treatment

recommended by the doctor was usually accepted without question. Now people are more cautious. They often wish to take responsibility for remaining healthy and find they can do this by following many of the principles of diet, exercise and treatment suggested by Chinese medicine. Many prefer not to use chemical drug treatments other than as a last resort.

The shock of the handicaps caused by *Thalidomide* in the 1960s, deaths attributed to *Opren* used for arthritis in the early 1980s and now in recent years questions surrounding other drugs such as *Steroids*, has caused distrust of the powerful drug companies. Other drugs such as the tranquillizer *Valium*, used extensively in the 1970s and thought to be non-addictive, were later found to have alarming side effects when people tried to come off them. Some people now see the drug companies as taking too little responsibility for their own mistakes and this causes great concern.

An interesting turn around is taking place. At one time complementary medicine was the last resort. Now Western treatment is often in this position. Many patients tell me that although they still trust their doctor's good intentions, they do not trust the drugs they are prescribed.

3 Since China opened up to the West in the 1970s, information about this system of medicine has become freely available. There is more literature and teaching accessible than ever before and many texts have been translated from Chinese into English, French, German and other languages. Other books have been written by Western authors. These books are often very inspiring and illuminating to the Western reader. Alongside these books there are also many colleges now open in the West. Here people can train in one of the Chinese medicines in three or four year courses.

4 One final reason for the popularity of Chinese medicine is that together with the other complementary medicines, it has received much publicity. Acupuncture and Chinese herbs are often in the news. Two surveys into complementary medicines were carried out by the consumer magazine *Which?*, in 1986 and 1995. Overall, 75 per cent of the 8,745 people who replied to the 1995 survey felt that their condition had been helped as a direct result of treatment and 83 per cent felt that their general sense of well being had improved. Of those who had acupuncture treatment 81 per cent said that they were satisfied with the results. Both surveys showed that overall people were pleased with the effects of their complementary treatments.

Chinese herbs have received much publicity for their beneficial effects in the treatment of skin conditions. One drug company is hoping to make a drug mimicking the main ingredients of the most common herbs used in the treatment of eczema. Although a Chinese herbalist will treat each patient individually and no one drug will deal with every type of eczema, it nevertheless shows that the drug companies are also noticing that Chinese herbs are effective.

Ear acupuncture is now used throughout the West in the treatment of drug dependence. Five 'detox' points on the ear have been found to be very successful in relieving craving for drugs.

These are only a few examples of the publicity given to Chinese medicine over recent years.

In this book, we will discuss each of the Chinese medicines in turn and hear from some of the patients who have used the different treatments. We will meet amongst others: Patricia, who cured her headaches by improving her diet; Margaret, whose skin problem went very suddenly when she had Chinese herbs;

Julia, who was able to get pregnant and is no longer anxious; Carol, who, with much thanks to acupuncture, has overcome her depression by regularly practising qigong; and Terry, whose back problem was cured by tui na massage.

These five therapies have formed the basis of Chinese medicine for thousands of years and are all linked. We will discuss the thread that links them in the first chapter of this book.

THE THEORY OF CHINESE MEDICINE
THE LINKING THREAD

Acupuncture, herbs, massage, diet and qigong – these treatments are all practised in their own special ways. An acupuncturist inserts a few fine needles into points, whilst a herbalist prescribes decoctions of herbs or pills, powders or tinctures. Qigong uses movement and exercise to create a better balance of health. A tui na masseur uses direct physical contact. Dietary therapy is advice about what to eat which the patient puts into practice at home. So what links these outwardly diverse treatments?

The linking thread is the theory of Chinese Medicine.

Whichever treatment a person chooses to have, the underlying theory comes from the same root. This forms the foundation for a unique diagnosis of each individual. Over the next few chapters we will be looking at these treatments and the theory that links them so that we can understand the basis of Chinese medicine.

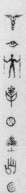

WHAT IS THE THEORY OF CHINESE MEDICINE?

There are three main components of the theory of Chinese medicine that are used in a diagnosis. Together they will enable the practitioner to find the exact energetic cause of a patient's complaint. They are *Yin and Yang*, *the Five Elements* and the *Vital Substances*. The *causes of disease* are described in the next chapter. Once a diagnosis has been formed, treatment will then work to re-establish the patient's health.

We will now examine each of these three components in turn. First, we will explore Yin and Yang, before looking at the Vital Substances and the Five Elements.

WHAT IS MEANT BY YIN AND YANG?

In order to diagnose the nature of a patient's problem a practitioner needs to understand and judge the relative balance of Yin and Yang in the individual. One of the oldest classics of Chinese medicine, *The Yellow Emperor's Classic of Internal Medicine* states:

To live in harmony with Yin and Yang means life.

To live against Yin and Yang means death.

To live in harmony with Yin and Yang will bring peace.

To live against Yin and Yang will bring chaos.

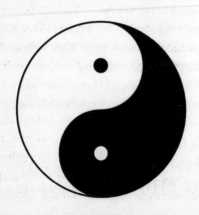

Yin and Yang symbol

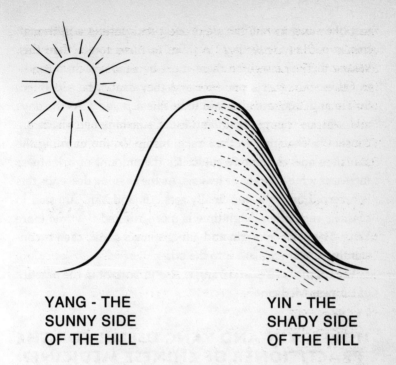

YANG - THE
SUNNY SIDE
OF THE HILL

YIN - THE
SHADY SIDE
OF THE HILL

Yin and Yang represent the two fundamental forces of the universe. The Chinese character for Yang means 'the sunny side of the hill' whilst for Yin the character depicts 'the shady side of the hill'. Chinese characters are an ideographic 'picture' which convey a vivid image of the meaning of the words they describe.

The Chinese define four main characteristics of Yin and Yang in order to describe their dynamic interaction. These are that 1) Yin and Yang are in opposition, 2) Yin and Yang are interdependent, 3) Yin and Yang consume each other, and 4) Yin and Yang transform into each other. The image of the sunny and shady sides of the hill depicts these four aspects very clearly.

Many people think of Yin and Yang as two *opposing* forces

4   just like sunshine and shade or light and darkness. Although this is partially true there is more to these forces than this. Where there is sunshine there must be shade, each is conditional on the other's presence and they cannot be separated. So Yin and Yang are also said to be *interdependent*. As the days and seasons change the quantities of sunshine and shade are constantly changing in their relationship. In the morning the sun rises and as the day continues the amount of brightness increases whilst the shade lessens. As the evening descends this is reversed until the sun finally sets. Yin and Yang are said to *consume* each other. Nighttime is more Yin and daytime more Yang. The balance of Yin and Yang is never static; each is constantly *transforming* one into the other.

The balance of Yin and Yang is also important in the practice of Chinese Medicine.

HOW IS YIN AND YANG USEFUL FOR THE PRACTITIONER OF CHINESE MEDICINE?

Each patient has her own particular balance of Yin and Yang. Yang is associated with *fire*; in other words it is dry, bright, hot, active and moving upwards and outwards. Yin can be characterized as associated with *water* as in a deep lake; in other words it is wet, dark and deep, cold and still.

When people become ill their balance of Yin and Yang will be affected. Sometimes they are hotter in temperature, overactive, feel drier in their bodies and may even become hotter tempered. In this case they have become more Yang in nature, the fire is starting to rage and is not held in check by the Yin. This may result in many different symptoms ranging from hot flushes to fevers, dark scanty urine, constipation and restlessness.

On the other hand some people feel the cold more, they may retain more body fluid, slow down and become very tired.

These people may have relatively too much Yin energy which is not held in check by their Yang. They may start to have symptoms of extreme chills, profuse pale urine, diarrhoea, lethargy or depression.

The fullness or deficiency of the body's Qi energy will determine how strongly the symptoms of a Yin/Yang imbalance will manifest. Fuller energy will create strong symptoms of 'full Yang' or 'full Yin'. Some people have very deficient energy and still manifest an imbalance. 'Yin deficiency' arises when a person's energy is deficient but there is relatively more Yang energy than Yin and this creates slight heat symptoms. 'Yang deficiency' arises in the opposite situation when there is relatively more Yin energy and less Yang, thus creating more symptoms of cold.

Some Yin and Yang Properties

YIN	YANG
Water	Fire
Cold	Heat
Wet	Dry
Interior	Exterior
Passive	Active
Slow	Rapid
Descending	Rising
Below	Above
Body	Head
Front	Back
Contraction	Expansion

The practitioner assesses the relative balance between Yin and Yang in each person. Knowing this, the therapist can then prescribe treatment to re-establish better equilibrium, thus restoring health.

Alongside the theory of Yin and Yang, the 'Vital Substances' are also important. We will now go on to explore what they are and how they affect diagnosis and treatment.

WHAT ARE THE VITAL SUBSTANCES?

The cells are the essential structure of the human body described in Western medicine and physiology is the science of the body's 'normal' functioning. The *Vital Substances* are their equivalent in Chinese medicine. They describe the main constituents of a person and the functioning of the Vital Substances could be described as 'Chinese physiology'.

The Vital Substances are the *Qi*, the *Jing Essence*, the *Blood*, the *Body-Fluids* and the *Shen* or *Mind-Spirit*. We'll now define each of these starting with Qi.

WHAT DO WE MEAN BY QI ENERGY?

Qi is the energy that underlies everything in the universe. Condensed it becomes matter, refined it becomes spirit. Everything that is living, moving and vibrating does so because Qi moves through it.

Qi inside our bodies is created from the combination of the food we eat and digest via our Stomach and Spleen and the air we breathe into our Lungs. In fact Chinese medicine considers Qi to be so important that an old Chinese text called the *Nan Jing* states:

Qi is the root of all human beings.

Qi creates all involuntary and voluntary movement such as the beating of our Hearts, the continuation of breathing while we sleep, as well as the assimilation of foods to nourish us, the ability to move our bodies from place to place or our thoughts

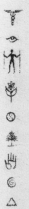

from subject to subject. Qi also protects us from illness and keeps our bodies warm.

To a practitioner of Chinese medicine the theory of Qi is important. If we looked through a microscope to try to see particles of Qi energy we would not find it, but the restoration of its balance is vital to recover a patient's health. If the Qi becomes deficient or blocked this will result in an inability to transform and transport our food and drink, an inability to keep warm, a lack of resistance to diseases and depleted energy.

A 50-year-old accountant came for treatment suffering from severe tiredness. He said, 'I find it hard to get up in the morning and often fall asleep in front of the television at night. I also feel extremely breathless just walking up the stairs.' On examination his practitioner found that his breathing was shallow and his chest very caved in and weak. He also had a weak and achy back which he said felt better when he put a heat pad on it. Many of his symptoms were due to 'Qi deficiency'. The Qi in his Lungs had become weakened after a chest infection, but a lack of exercise coupled with sitting at his desk in a bad posture was making the deficiency worse. He was told to exercise more and take breaks from his desk work as well as having other Chinese treatments.

Besides diagnosing the functioning of a person's Qi the practitioner also examines the state of the Blood which flows with the Qi in the body.

WHAT DOES THE TERM 'BLOOD' MEAN IN CHINESE MEDICINE?

To many of us the question 'What is Blood?' seems like a silly question. We all know that it is the red stuff that flows through our arteries and veins! In the practice of Chinese medicine, however, the Blood is described by its function rather than by what it is.

8   The term *Blood* to a practitioner of Chinese medicine means the fluid that nourishes and moisturizes the body. It also houses the *Shen* or Mind-Spirit (see later in this chapter). The symptoms of Blood 'deficiency' are very commonly seen by practitioners of Chinese medicine. They may be caused by heavy bleeding and are especially common in women who have heavy periods or lose a lot of Blood whilst giving birth, but can also be caused by a diet lacking in protein or by excessive anxiety.

Symptoms of 'Blood deficiency' include frequent pins and needles or cramps due to malnourishment of the muscles and tendons, dry skin and brittle nails due to lack of moistening of the skin, and constant anxiety, poor memory and lack of concentration due to the Blood not 'housing' the Shen. A person who is Blood deficient will also often have a dull-pale complexion.

Blood can also stagnate causing extreme pain and even fixed masses such as fibroids or lumps, or it can become overheated causing bleeding symptoms such as uterine haemorrhage or nosebleeds.

When people have problems with their Blood a practitioner may use herbs or other Chinese treatments to create a better state of health. Often the patient can help the healing process by making dietary changes especially by adding more protein to the diet (see page 122).

The state of a patient's Qi and Blood are dependent on the underlying constitution which we will consider next.

WHAT IS 'JING' AND HOW IS IT IMPORTANT TO OUR HEALTH?

We inherit our Jing Essence from our parents. The strength of it decides the robustness of our constitution. Jing is stored in the kidneys and allows us to develop from childhood to adulthood and then into old age. Children reach puberty, then mature until they can conceive and have children. At the end of their fertile lives women go through the menopause and stop menstruating. The ability to move through these different stages and cycles of our lives is due to the Jing.

The Jing that we inherit at birth is the quantity that we have for the rest of our lives. Some people are frail and weak from birth or have slightly slower mental or physical development than usual. Although they may be slightly 'Jing deficient', if they conserve their energy carefully they can live long and happy lives. Some illnesses which we term 'congenital' illnesses may also be due to deficient Jing.

Most of us have an average amount of Jing. There is no situation in which people have too much Jing – those people with exceptionally strong constitutions are just called lucky!

As we start to age, greying hair, falling teeth and failing memories are all signs that the Jing is becoming depleted. Aging is a natural process but the more care we put into looking after our overall health the better we conserve our Jing later in life. Our constitutional strength is difficult to change so extreme Jing deficiencies can be hard to treat. Treatment on the Kidneys which store the Jing can, however, prevent problems from developing. Many qigong practitioners say that regular practise of qigong will conserve Jing and some say it can even build it up.

The next substance we will discuss is our Body Fluids which must flow smoothly and be in good supply to retain good health.

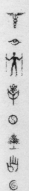

WHAT ARE OUR BODY FLUIDS AND HOW IMPORTANT ARE THEY TO A PRACTITIONER OF CHINESE MEDICINE?

'Jin Ye' are the words used in Chinese medicine for all the fluids in the body. The Jin body fluids are light and watery and are at the exterior of our body. These nourish the skin and muscles and come out as sweat and also saliva and mucus. The fluids that are heavier and more inside our bodies, are called Ye. The Ye moisturize the joints, brain, the spine and bone marrow.

If the Body Fluids become deficient we dehydrate, if they get stuck and are not moving smoothly around the body, they may be retained. When women get heavy thighs or men the formation of a paunch this can be due to stuck body fluids which the Chinese call 'Damp'. Oedema in the body is also due to retained body fluids. Treatment on the Spleen can be a very important way of moving body fluids as the Spleen transforms and transports everything in the body. If the Body Fluids are stuck this can obstruct the free movement of the Qi and Blood in the body. The Body Fluids are the most 'substantial' of all of the Substances in the body; this is in contrast to the Shen which is the most 'insubstantial'.

WHAT IS OUR SHEN AND WHERE IS IT?

Our *Shen* could be said to be a very rarefied form of Qi but it could also be called our very spirit itself. It is housed in the Heart by the Blood. The Shen is said to be so refined and light that it needs the Blood which is a heavier substance to keep it settled in place. If our Blood is weakened our Shen can become what is called 'disturbed' and we become anxious, jumpy, lacking in concentration and possibly have difficulty sleeping. A strong and calm Shen gives us the ability to sleep well, to think clearly, have a good memory and a strong sense of purpose in our lives. It will also show itself by a bright sparkle in the eye.

The Shen, the Qi and the Jing are called 'the Three Treasures'. Together they are the basis of our health. The Chinese will often use the term 'Jingshen' as a short-hand term for vitality or vigour indicating their understanding that good constitution and a strong spirit are the basis of a healthy life.

Alongside Yin and Yang and the Vital Substances, a knowledge of the Five Elements and their twelve organs is important in diagnosis so that we can understand any imbalance in an individual.

WHAT ARE THE FIVE ELEMENTS?

The Chinese character for an element is 'xing' and this depicts something that is a moving force, a phase, or something transforming or changing. The Five Elements can be said to be five dynamic qualities that are all interacting with each other and which ultimately correspond with everything in the universe.

The names of the Five Elements are Wood, Fire, Earth, Metal and Water. These Elements are connected with many different qualities. Each resonates with a season, a climate, a taste, a colour, a sound, an emotion, an odour, a movement, a sense organ and a body part as well as having many other associations. They are also each linked with two different internal organs, a Yang organ and a Yin organ. The Water Element, for example, is related to the Bladder and the Kidney, both of which are associated with the assimilation of water in our bodies. The Earth element is connected with the Stomach and Spleen. Food grows on the earth so there is an obvious relationship between these organs and this Element.

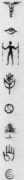

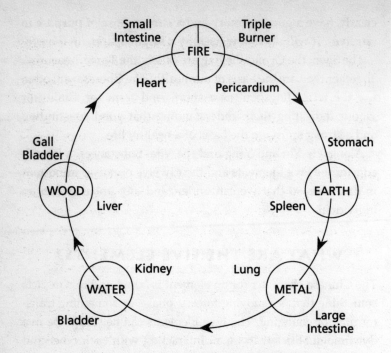

The Five Elements and the associated organs

HOW ARE THE FIVE ELEMENTS USED IN DIAGNOSIS?

The Five Elements are interconnected and each promotes the next. They are often depicted as joining together in a clockwise moving circle (see diagram). Because of this interconnectedness, when one of the organs and its associated Element is out of balance the other Elements are also affected. This imbalance will manifest in the individual with many different signs and symptoms. It may show in the facial colour, the sound of the voice, a slight change in the emotional state as well as disharmony in the functioning of the connected organs.

For example, a female patient in her late twenties is treated on her Liver and Gall Bladder. These organs are associated with the Wood Element. She complains, 'I often feel extremely angry, especially before my period starts.' She also shows a blue-green colour on her face around her mouth and by the side of her eyes and she speaks with a slightly shouting voice tone. Her other premenstrual symptoms include tenderness and slight swelling of her breasts and a bloated abdomen. These are all signs and symptoms associated with the Wood Element. One of the functions of the Liver is to ensure that the energy is flowing smoothly in the person. If it is not, it will bring about symptoms such as bloating, because the energy is stagnating. The cause of this stagnation is often frustration and anger. A person who is angry holds her muscles very tensely and can prevent the energy from flowing smoothly and freely in the body.

Five Element associations

	WOOD	FIRE	EARTH	METAL	WATER
Yin Organ	Liver	Heart Pericardium	Spleen	Lung	Kidney
Yang Organ	Gall bladder	Small intestine Triple burner	Stomach	Large Intestine	Bladder
Colour	Blue-green	Red	Yellow	White	Blue-black
Sound	Shout	Laugh	Sing	Weep	Groan
Emotion	Anger	Joy	Worry/ Sympathy	Grief	Fear
Odour	Rancid	Scorched	Fragrant	Rotten	Putrid
Season	Spring	Summer	Late summer	Autumn	Winter
Climate	Wind	Heat	Damp	Dryness	Cold
Tastes	Sour	Bitter	Sweet	Pungent	Salty
Body Parts	Tendons	Blood and blood vessels	Muscles and flesh	Skin and fascia	Bone and marrow
Movements	Expansion outwards	Upward movement	Neutrality and stability	Contraction inwards	Downward movement

HOW ARE THE ORGANS USED IN DIAGNOSIS AND TREATMENT?

The organs are also called the 'Zang-Fu'. *Zang* means a Yin organ and *Fu* means a Yang organ. These have a far wider scope of functioning and influence than the purely physiological function described in the West. The Zang organs each have a main use linked with one of the Vital Substances. They also are connected to a sense organ, and have an associated spiritual aspect.

Major functions of the yin organs

ORGAN	ASSOCIATED SUBSTANCE	SENSE ORGAN	SPIRITUAL ASPECT
Heart	Makes blood. Governs Blood which is pumped around the body. Houses the Shen or Mind-Spirit	Tongue	Mind-Spirit creates ability to sleep, think clearly and to have a good memory
Liver	Creates 'free flowing' of Qi. Stores the Blood	Eye	Imparts vision and the ability to make clear future plans
Lung	Governs Qi and respiration	Nose	Animates the body and creates instinctive reactions
Spleen	Makes and controls Blood and keeps it in Blood vessels. Transforms and transports food and fluid	Mouth	Creates intention and ability to draw thoughts into form
Kidney	Stores Jing or Essence. Transports and transforms Body Fluids	Ear	Creates drive and willpower

As well as these organs there are two other functions which are unknown in Western physiology. These are the Pericardium and the Triple Burner. The Pericardium has a function of protecting the Heart from emotional upsets and 'knocks'. When we feel vulnerable and are easily hurt this may be due to imbalance in the functioning of this 'Heart Protector'. The Pericardium also protects us from external 'attacks' such as infections.

The Triple Burner has the purpose of harmonizing the organs and ensuring the safe passage of energy and fluids throughout our bodies. Malfunctioning can cause Qi or Body Fluids to become blocked in our systems.

If one of these organs or functions becomes imbalanced the associated Substance, sense organ or spiritual aspect can also become affected and its positive effects will no longer manifest. For instance, if the Liver is in disharmony we will have symptoms caused by stagnation of the free flow of our energy such as the premenstrual symptoms described in the previous patient. Besides this we may also have difficulty making future plans and decisions and thus have little direction in our lives. As the imbalanced organ is treated, symptoms will change in many ways. This indicates that the functioning of our body, mind and spirit has become more harmonized.

Yin and Yang, the Five Elements and the Vital Substances form the basis of the diagnosis made by a practitioner of Chinese medicine. Before looking more closely at how they are used together, we will examine another essential part of the theory of Chinese medicine – the causes of disease and how the Chinese view good health.

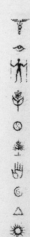

HOW DISEASE ARISES
THE ART OF STAYING HEALTHY

S ome people think that to be healthy is simply to be without an illness and if they have no signs and symptoms of disease they must be well. The Chinese view health differently. Being well is a very positive state, one in which we feel vibrant, vital and energetic and are happy to be alive. Health is something that is experienced at every level of our being, both physically and in our spirit.

Pattie, a patient, explains how she understood health before she had treatment:

'I was a nurse and can remember walking to work on the wards and wondering about my own health. I'd think, 'I'm physically healthy, my mind is clear and I've got nothing wrong with me. So why do I feel so unwell?' I felt desperately low in energy. I was like a robot getting through life but not living it. I never went to the doctor as there was nothing I could say was wrong.

'A few years later I developed a minor rash. A friend told me about Chinese medicine and I decided to try it. I'm so glad I went for treatment. My rash cleared very quickly but more importantly I felt much better. My spirits lifted and I felt positively well. My life became enjoyable and I realized that this really was good health. What I'd experienced before was a "lack of illness".'

In order to understand how to become healthy, first we need to ask how disease arises.

SO HOW DOES DISEASE COME ABOUT?

The Chinese divide the causes of disease into three main areas. The first are 'Internal' causes, which are illnesses caused by emotions. The second are the 'External' causes which are climatic conditions. The third are 'Miscellaneous' causes; these cover constitution, diet, exercise, rest, sexual behaviour and trauma. We'll now look at each of these in turn. First, the 'Internal' causes.

WHAT ARE THE INTERNAL CAUSES OF DISEASE?

The Internal causes of disease have only recently been given recognition in our Western society. It is astonishing that the Chinese wrote about them in their texts thousands of years ago when they identified the impact of emotional factors on physical health.

The Internal causes of disease are *anger*, *sadness*, *worry*, *fear*, *joy*, *grief*, *pensiveness* and *shock*. Other emotions are seen as an extension or a combination of these seven. To express these emotions appropriately is a normal and healthy response to the many situations we encounter in daily life. For example, we will feel afraid when we are threatened, angry if we are let down, or sadness when we lose someone or something important to us.

HOW DO EMOTIONS CAUSE DISEASE?

Emotions only cause disease when they are intense or prolonged or if they are not expressed or acknowledged over a long period of time. Sometimes they start from conditions which began in our childhood when we were unable to change our circumstances.

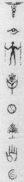

We may have been affected by situations involving parents, siblings, teachers or schoolmates. Occasionally these are sudden events such as the loss of a parent or friend. At other times they are more gradual in onset such as continual rejection by an important person which may result in a loss of self-esteem and confidence. Later these incidents and patterns from so long ago may begin to affect our health and well-being.

A female patient now in her thirties came for treatment complaining, 'I often feel sick and have loose bowels. I'm also a worrier, especially about my daughter.' She had become obsessional that something terrible would happen to the seven year old. On taking her case history it became apparent that these problems were rooted in her early childhood when her mother had a serious accident. The patient as a child had no one to turn to for support and she worried continually that her mother would die. Treatment on her Stomach and Spleen Qi helped both her body and her mind. She became less anxious for her daughter's well-being as well as more settled in her stomach and bowels. Digestion is a process of assimilation both physically and mentally.

Intense emotions in the present can also take their toll on our health. We may feel continuously worried, anxious or frustrated in a situation at work or at home. Sometimes we get through these events unscathed. At other times we do not. A male patient in his early twenties came for acupuncture treatment having had a harrowing week at work. 'My boss has been putting too much pressure on me and expecting me to meet impossible deadlines,' he raged. Treatment soothed his energy which had become imbalanced by his frustration. He immediately felt better and consequently found that he was able to sort out the matter with his boss.

At times it is obvious that the cause of a patient's illness is an Internal one but it is unclear exactly which emotions or events

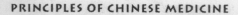

brought it about. It is not necessary to know this and the patient can still be treated successfully.

Many illnesses are originally caused by an Internal factor. This may have weakened the person and made her more vulnerable to the external, climatic causes of disease which we will discuss next.

HOW CAN EXTERNAL CONDITIONS CAUSE DISEASE?

Climatic conditions as a cause of disease are written about in texts from as far back as 3,000 years ago. The main climatic conditions are *Wind, Cold, Damp, Heat* and *Dryness*. Different climatic conditions are appropriate during each season and we usually adapt to them as they come and go. Summer should be hot and winter should be cold. The springtime brings a warming up after the cold of winter and there is a natural cooling down again in the autumn.

Extremes of weather such as a very cold winter or unseasonal weather such as a warm spell in winter make us more vulnerable to the effects of that climatic condition and consequently to becoming ill.

Sometimes we create these 'unusual seasonal conditions' for ourselves! A young female patient went on a wonderful hot winter holiday abroad over Christmas and was surprised to have a terrible cold on her return. This was due to her system being unable to adapt from the warm climate abroad to the English winter on coming home. 'I felt so healthy while I was away,' she commented after the cold had gone, 'now I feel worse than before I went.'

People whose underlying energy is weak are more vulnerable to the effects of climatic conditions than those who have a strong constitution and never get sick. For example, as people

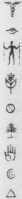

age they generally grow more fragile. During an exceptionally cold winter we may worry about our older relatives and friends and encourage them to keep warm, knowing that the cold brings greater danger of hypothermia and other illnesses.

Below is a list of these External pathogenic factors and the kinds of symptoms they might cause if they affect us.

The external causes of diseases

EXTERNAL PATHOGEN AND ITS NATURE	AREAS OF SYMPTOMS CREATED	EXAMPLES OF ILLNESSES
Wind arises suddenly, changes rapidly, has an upward and outward movement and makes things shake and sway.	Symptoms that come on suddenly, constantly change or move around. Symptoms where there is shaking or sudden movement. Symptoms at the top of or outside the body.	Head colds and flus, joint pains that move around, epilepsy, strokes, Parkinson's disease, some skin conditions.
Damp is sticky and lingering. Heavy and dirty.	Symptoms that do not change easily. Symptoms of heaviness or obstruction. Oozing and discharges.	Heavy or muzzy head, stiff or heavy limbs, bloated abdomen, vaginal discharge, pus-filled spots, tiredness.
Cold impairs moving and warming in the body. It contracts tissues and obstructs circulation causing pain.	Symptoms of biting and sharp pain which are relieved by warmth and made worse by cold. Contraction of tendons.	Loose bowels, period pains, stomach pains, cold hands and feet, frostbite, painful joints.
Heat has an upward direction, depletes the energy, dries up body fluids. Disturbs the spirit.	Feels hot, body parts red, intense thirst, bitter taste, profuse bleeding, dark scanty urine.	Sore throat, cystitis, constipation, red eyes, mania, restlessness.
Dryness injures blood, dries body fluids.	Dry throat, dry skin, dry mouth, dry stools, dry lips, scanty urination.	Some skin problems, constipation, chest conditions.

Besides helping a patient by using appropriate treatment, a practitioner can advise patients of ways in which they can protect themselves from adverse climatic conditions and avoid succumbing to their effects. Some of these ways are listed below. We can see that External causes can be primary reasons for illness occurring. There are other significant causes known as the Miscellaneous causes of disease.

Some Golden Rules to Protect Ourselves From External Conditions

WIND

Wrap up against the windy weather especially around the neck. Keep covered if the temperature changes when returning from sunny holidays abroad or going in and out of overheated or air-conditioned shops. Don't sleep or stand in front of a fan or in a draft. These could cause headaches or lower resistance to colds or influenza.

COLD

Don't walk around with no shoes on especially on cold floors as this could cause period pain or even infertility. Keep the midriff covered to avoid stomach pain and the back covered to prevent backaches.

DAMP

If you live in a damp house buy a dehumidifier to avoid symptoms such as a muzzy head, tiredness or poor concentration. Dry yourself properly after bathing or swimming to avoid joint pains.

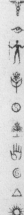

HEAT

Beware of staying out in the sun for too long to avoid over-heating or heat stroke. Don't sleep with your head towards a nearby radiator or oven in order to prevent headaches, red eyes and a bad temper.

DRYNESS

If staying in a centrally-heated environment, moisten the atmosphere with a bowl of water to avoid dry cough, dry skin or a dry throat.

WHAT DO WE MEAN BY THE MISCELLANEOUS CAUSES OF DISEASE?

The Miscellaneous causes of disease are ones that are neither External to our bodies as are climatic conditions, nor Internal as are emotions. Literally translated from Chinese these are called 'not internal and not external' causes of disease. They cover areas such as constitution, overwork and fatigue, exercise, sex, diet and trauma.

It is important not to underestimate the significance of a healthy, regular diet in relation to our health. This is covered in much greater detail in chapter 8 on 'Dietetics'. Jing Essence, the basis of our constitution has already been described in chapter 1.

We will now take a brief look at the other Miscellaneous causes of disease.

HOW DO BALANCED AMOUNTS OF WORK AND REST PREVENT DISEASE?

The issue of how much we *work* and how much we *rest* is an important one in today's society. Nowadays pressure is often put on people to work very hard and to return to work quickly after they have been ill. The word 'convalescence' is almost unheard of these days in relation to time spent recovering from an illness. Often people with colds and other infections say, 'Oh, don't worry, I'll work right through it', or if they do have time off, feel guilty for taking more than the bare minimum.

There is a strong case for people taking an extra day or two to recover and throw off their illness completely. If people do not allow themselves to fully recover, the infection can remain latent in their bodies. It can then return in the form of what is often called a 'post-viral syndrome'. Many post-viral syndromes are the result of a combination of continual overwork and a lack of convalescence after infection. A person then often feels continually depleted and run down and is unable to recover from the illness at all. Post-viral syndromes often last for many years and all for the sake of an extra few days' rest! As one patient observed, 'I had rested a little after being ill, but then I went back to work. I worked much too hard – and then it was too late. All my energy had gone and I didn't recover for many years.'

HOW CAN EXERCISE BENEFIT MY HEALTH?

The last 50 years have also seen a considerable decrease in the amount of natural exercise we get. The use of cars has reduced the quantity of walking we do. Household gadgets such as washing machines and vacuum cleaners have lessened the amount of exercise we would naturally get around the house

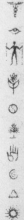

(thank goodness!). Many children spend less time in the rough and tumble of the playground as they are happy to play on their computers instead – a worrying trend.

Few of us want to be without our labour-saving devices but the resulting effect on our lifestyle means that we need to find alternative ways of exercising and remaining healthy. A friend of mine recently, told me, 'I've started to cycle to work instead of driving as I was beginning to feel like a couch potato. Surprisingly, I have much more energy even though I'm exerting myself more and I've also lost some weight.'

Too much exercise can be just as detrimental as too little. A friend who once obsessively exercised observed, 'I felt great while I was out running. Then I realized my good intentions had backfired on me. I was wearing myself out and felt completely drained the rest of the time.'

We need to be realistic about the amount of exercise we get so that we can remain healthy. A balanced amount of work and rest combined with exercise is still as important as it was 50 years ago.

We will now focus on two other important miscellaneous causes of disease which are sexual behaviour and trauma.

IN WHAT WAY CAN SEX BECOME A CAUSE OF DISEASE?

The Chinese recognized that too much sex can be a cause of disease. They warned that this is especially important for men rather than women. Men can wear out their Kidney energy if they ejaculate too much. This can result in possible back problems, tiredness and premature ageing. The issue of what exactly is too much sex, has been much debated in many texts throughout Chinese history!

However much we agree or disagree with this Chinese

notion of too much sex, there are some clear and sensible guidelines we can follow. Young adults have more energy for sex than older people and can therefore afford to be more sexually active in their younger years. We can also have more sex in the summer when we naturally tend to be more active, than in the winter when it is more normal for us to do less. The Chinese also advise less sex if we are ill as we need to conserve our strength in order to regain our health.

Of course there is a natural balance between too much and too little sex. Too little sex can lead to much frustration and resentment, also possibly causing illness. In general the 'right' amount of sex could be said to be as much as satisfies each couple and is part of a fulfilling relationship for them both.

HOW IS PHYSICAL TRAUMA A CAUSE OF DISEASE?

Any accident or injury can be a cause of later disease in the part of the body involved. Western doctors tell us that a broken bone or a joint strain can be the site of 'arthritic changes' occurring later on in life. If this happens a patient experiences pain, stiffness, swelling, heat or limitation of movement in the area that was injured a long time previously. A practitioner of Chinese medicine would say that this injury left the joint vulnerable to Wind, Cold or Damp entering it or to Heat being formed inside the joint.

Damp in a joint tends to cause stiffness and swelling, as Damp is said to be sticky and lingering. Wind causes pain that comes and goes and moves from place to place, just like the wind in nature. Cold contracts the tendons and causes sharp pain like the pain in the fingers caused by holding a snowball in the hand for too long. Heat in a joint causes the redness, swelling and pain that we experience when there is

26   inflammation in the body. These pathogens entering the joints after injury can often be eliminated by using Chinese treatments of herbs, acupuncture, tui na massage or qigong.

The Causes of Disease

EXTERNAL
Wind, Cold, Damp, Dryness, Heat.

INTERNAL
Anger, Fear, Grief, Joy, Worry, Pensiveness, Shock.

MISCELLANEOUS
Constitution, Overwork and Fatigue, Exercise, Diet, Sex, Trauma.

DO I HAVE TO KNOW THE CAUSE OF MY PROBLEM TO BE TREATED FOR IT?

For most people the causes of their problems are a combination of Internal, External and Miscellaneous factors. Many people are unaware of what have been the specific reasons behind their sickness. The practitioner will diagnose the patient's condition so that she can understand and treat the underlying energetic imbalance. Treatment can then successfully clear the symptoms.

A middle-aged female patient, for instance, came for treatment having been affected by a 'virus' for a number of weeks. She said, 'I'm aching all over and I'm really tired. I also have loose bowels and I'm really bloated in my stomach.' These were all symptoms of an External 'attack' of Dampness. She received herbs and acupuncture treatment which cleared it, but could not remember any time when she had been in Damp conditions which could have precipitated the condition.

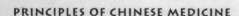

Other illnesses may have taken root in early childhood and patients often don't know the exact cause of the resulting problems. In spite of this, patients can still be treated successfully. Sometimes the cause of the condition becomes clearer and resolves itself as treatment progresses.

HOW ARE THE CAUSES OF DISEASE USED IN DIAGNOSIS AND TREATMENT?

Although it is not always necessary to understand the origin of a disease in order to cure it, it can be helpful to know the main reasons why diseases have occurred, especially when they have arisen due to a person's living habits. Patients may consider whether they are eating properly, getting enough rest and exercise or whether they need to work less. This may help them to understand the problems that brought about their illness and to make lifestyle changes which could help them to become healthier.

Not everyone finds it easy to make immediate shifts in their lifestyle even if they would be healthier as a result. They can, however, gain more insight into why they have become ill and strive towards a healthier balance. The Chinese believe that the best recipe for health is a balanced lifestyle and avoiding extremes in anything we do. We can all use this as a rule of thumb when considering our health needs.

Next we will consider how the theories of Chinese medicine that we have discussed in the first two chapters are put together to form a diagnosis.

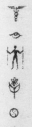

PUTTING IT ALL TOGETHER

DIAGNOSIS IN CHINESE MEDICINE

Yin and Yang, *the Five Elements* and *the Vital Substances*, together with *the causes of disease* are the foundation of an accurate diagnosis for each individual. So what is this diagnosis like for the patient?

Here are some comments people have made about their diagnosis: 'I remember feeling as if I'd had a huge burden lifted from me and I appreciated that the practitioner had the time to listen to me.' 'It was absolutely wonderful, I was asked questions nobody had asked me before. I also got reassurance that I could be helped.' 'It was so thorough that I had the opportunity to say whatever I wanted not just about my physical health but about how I was feeling too.'

HOW LONG WILL THE DIAGNOSIS TAKE?

Practitioners of acupuncture, herbs or tui na all wish to help people to become healthier. Most have a strong sense of vocation and a great desire to assist people to overcome their illnesses and enjoy a better quality of life. People may be nervous when they go for a diagnosis and are surprised by the amount of time and personal care they are given by the practitioner.

A full diagnosis will usually take anything from one to two

hours. This will vary according to the practitioner, the type of treatment and the needs of the patient. Patients often feel that they have established a good rapport with their practitioner during this consultation and that the act of talking through their problems is in itself very helpful in understanding their own health.

WHAT SHOULD I EXPECT AT THE DIAGNOSIS?

Practitioners will ask their patients why they have come for treatment and many other details about their problems. They will ask questions which will vary from 'How well do you sleep at night?' or 'How is your appetite?' to 'Are there any frustrations or difficulties that you are currently having in your life?' or 'What do you do in your spare time?' These questions and many more are all relevant to the patient's health.

Practitioners may also palpate different areas of the body to test for sensitivity or pain or to feel for temperature, and they may observe other signs such as facial colour. The face may show different coloured 'hues' such as green if the Liver and Gall Bladder are out of balance or blue-black if the Kidney and Bladder are deficient.

Practitioners will also pay attention to the patient's posture and will even notice the sparkle in the eye which will tell them about the state of the patient's 'spirit'. They will also feel the patient's pulse and look at the tongue. These are two important areas of a diagnosis which we will now explore in more detail.

HOW DOES A PRACTITIONER DIAGNOSE USING THE PULSES?

The practitioner feels twelve pulses at both wrists in order to diagnose the state of the patient's Qi and Blood as well as the

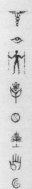

condition of both the Yin and Yang organs. The pulse is felt with three fingers along the radial artery and each position corresponds to one of the 12 organs.

The 12 pulse positions

	LEFT WRIST		RIGHT WRIST	
	YANG ORGAN	YIN ORGAN	YIN ORGAN	YANG ORGAN
1st position	Small intestine	Heart	Lung	Large intestine
2nd position	Gall bladder	Liver	Spleen	Stomach
3rd position	Bladder	Kidney (Yin)	Pericardium kidney (Yang)	Triple burner

There are many different qualities that can be felt on the pulses and these correspond to the patient's own energy balance. For example, when a person has an illness deep inside the body the pulse will feel deep down or be 'sinking'. If there is a pathogen such as 'Wind' invading the Lungs causing a common cold the pulses will 'float' or feel more superficial as this illness is at a superficial level of the body. In this case the position of the Lung is often the most affected.

The pulses also have an overall strength or depletion according to the patient's general energy balance and according to which organs are affected. If a person feels 'uptight' and angry she will often have a stretched tight feeling on the pulse known as a 'wiry' pulse or if there is a depletion of the blood the pulse will feel thin as there is less blood to fill up the blood vessels.

Altogether there are 28 qualities that can be felt on the pulse and patients will often have more than one quality manifesting. Pulse diagnosis is a skill that a practitioner of Chinese medicine develops over a lifetime. It is very different from pulse diagnosis used in modern Western medicine. Both feel the pulse at the radial artery but the Western doctor or nurse counts the pulse rate only. Practitioners of Chinese medicine will notice the rate but will also feel the whole range of other qualities which are also present.

WHAT IS TONGUE DIAGNOSIS?

The colour, shape, moisture, movement, coating and areas of the tongue are used to diagnose the state of our internal organs. Disharmony will often show on the tongue before symptoms start to make themselves felt. A healthy tongue will be pale red in colour, fairly moist, fit snugly into the mouth and have a thin white coating. Sometimes the tongue looks redder than normal. This shows the presence of heat whilst a pale tongue may indicate cold. The tongue is filled with Blood so it will also naturally become paler when Blood is deficient.

A tongue can become swollen. This is often due to excess Body Fluids such as 'Damp' being stuck in the body or the Yang energy becoming deficient so that the body becomes cold and Body Fluids don't move. A thin tongue body can mean a lack of Body Fluids.

Each area of the tongue corresponds to a different organ in the body. These areas can be wet or dry, thin or swollen, pale or

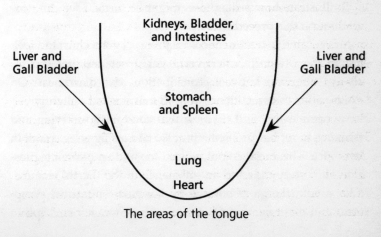

Kidneys, Bladder, and Intestines

Liver and Gall Bladder

Liver and Gall Bladder

Stomach and Spleen

Lung

Heart

The areas of the tongue

PRINCIPLES OF CHINESE MEDICINE

red according to which organ of the body is out of balance. For instance, red sides of the tongue can mean Heat in the Liver and Gall Bladder, red in the centre can mean Heat in the Stomach or red at the tongue tip can mean Heat in the Heart. Sometimes the tongue has red 'spots' at the tip indicating a tendency to become easily emotionally upset.

HOW IS THE THEORY OF CHINESE MEDICINE USED TO CREATE A DIAGNOSIS?

During the diagnosis the practitioner has gathered together information about the patient's signs and symptoms, has observed the tongue and the facial colour and felt the pulses on the wrist. The practitioner is now ready to make a diagnosis.

Knowledge of Yin and Yang, the Five Elements and the Vital Substances can lead to a simple yet elegant diagnosis which can pinpoint the cause of the patient's problem very accurately while at the same time continuing to view the patient holistically. The cause of the imbalance might be an Internal, an External or a Miscellaneous cause of disease.

To illustrate how a diagnosis might be formed we can now go through this procedure step by step.

Mrs G came to treatment complaining, 'I get a churning feeling in my Stomach whenever I get upset and my Bowels always alternate between constipation and diarrhoea.' On examination the practitioner noticed that she had a slightly yellowy complexion, and that she was constantly worrying and thinking about her problem. She also had a sing-song sound in her voice. This facial colour, voice tone and emotional expression all corresponded to an imbalance in the 'Earth' element. This was further corroborated by her gastro-intestinal symptoms and other symptoms involving her Stomach and Spleen such as a poor appetite, weakness in her limbs and a bloating feeling after eating. The Qi of the Spleen was weak. The churning feeling came and went according to the severity of her emotional state as did the constipation and diarrhoea. The diagnosis revealed that the Stomach and Spleen of the Earth element were the primary cause of her problems but that her Liver was also involved, creating symptoms that came and went and further affected her Stomach and Spleen. The diagnosis was Liver Qi 'invades' the Stomach and Spleen. This was treated by acupuncture and Chinese herbs.

Mrs S came to her practitioner complaining, 'I get terrible menopausal hot flushes. They especially wake me at night.' Upon examination the practitioner noticed that she had a blue-black facial colour especially around her eyes although she also had a red face caused by the heat. She had a monotone sound in her voice, and she was very fearful and anxious. These symptoms were connected to the Water Element which was out of balance and was affecting her Bladder and Kidney organs. This was her primary imbalance. Her Heart energy was also affected. This was indicated by symptoms such as palpitations, poor sleep and restlessness which were all symptoms connected with the Heart. The practitioner diagnosed that the Heart did not have enough 'Yin' energy and this was causing symptoms of too much Heat. The diagnosis was Kidney and Heart Yin deficiency which was rebalanced using different forms of Chinese medicine.

Whether the patient's condition is caused by 'Liver Qi invades the Stomach and Spleen' or 'Heart and Kidney Yin deficiency', the same diagnosis will be made by a practitioner of any branch of Chinese medicine.

Having understood the basis of Chinese medical theory we can now go on to examine each of these treatments in turn. We will start with acupuncture and moxibustion.

ACUPUNCTURE AND MOXIBUSTION
BALANCING YOUR ENERGY

A cupuncture was the first of the traditional Chinese treatments to hit the headlines in the West. It was introduced in France by Georges Soulie de Morant, a French diplomat. He was inspired by seeing acupuncture used successfully to treat people with cholera – a certain killer at that time. Having witnessed its miraculous healing powers, he knew he had to learn its secrets so that others could experience them too. He started teaching acupuncture in 1939 and it has been practised in Europe ever since that time.

It was when President Nixon visited China in 1972, however, that acupuncture really took off. The sight of fully-conscious Chinese patients chatting to nurses while undergoing major surgery had a profound influence on people. It was obviously not faked and such a strange form of treatment captured the imagination of both the American and the English public. The West's romance with Chinese Medicine had begun.

Whilst acupuncture anaesthesia and pain relief were generally accepted, it is only recently that its many other uses have become apparent.

Although most people have now heard about acupuncture they frequently don't know much about it. When I asked people who'd never had acupuncture, 'What do you think acupuncture is?', these were some of the replies I was given. 'It's the awful stuff when they stick needles in you!' 'It's lots of needles going in you, urgh.' 'It's a needle thing – scary stuff!' Some people were more positive, 'It's the use of needles to cure various ailments.' 'I wouldn't have it myself but I've heard favourable reports from people.' 'My mum had it and she got much better.' Although people knew it involved the use of needles many people associated acupuncture with something that was scary and painful rather than with something healing and calming.

The purpose of this chapter is to give you an objective look at acupuncture treatment and answer the questions most frequently asked about it.

WHAT ARE ACUPUNCTURE AND MOXIBUSTION?

The word *acupuncture* has its roots in Latin. The Latin word *acus* means a needle, so acupuncture means 'to puncture with a needle'.

Acupuncturists practise their art with a few fine needles, inserting them into points on the body. These points are located and join together in 'channels' or 'meridians' along which Qi flows. The points used in treatment are carefully chosen by the practitioner to disperse any blockages and to bring the patient's Qi into balance. The more this balance is achieved, the healthier the patient becomes.

When we talk about 'acupuncture treatment' in the West we usually mean acupuncture and moxibustion. Both treatments have been used together throughout Chinese history. The Chinese words for these treatments are *Zhen* and *Jiu*. *Zhen* means acupuncture and *Jiu* means moxibustion.

Moxibustion is the burning of a herb close to the body. This herb *Artemesia vulgaris latiflora* is similar to our native mug-

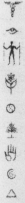

wort. 'Moxa' as it is often called, is used alongside needles to warm our Qi when we are too cold and also to nourish and regulate our Qi in a more general sense. Historically it was first used in the more northern parts of China where it is colder.

We'll discuss moxa and needles in greater detail later in this chapter. First, let's find out more about the channels and points which are used in treatment.

WHAT ARE THE 'MERIDIANS' OR 'CHANNELS'?

The channels or meridians are lines of Qi running throughout our bodies. These meridians form a network which the Chinese have compared to an irrigation system. The Chinese have used irrigation systems to nourish and water the land for thousands of years. These systems break down if they are neglected. The water in the ditches might dry up and the surrounding areas are starved of nourishment.

Likewise, our meridian system can become blocked or depleted causing an imbalance in the Qi and eventually illness. Acupuncture lets the Qi flow freely again, clearing blockages and nourishing the Qi. This in turn restores our health.

WHERE ARE THE MERIDIANS AND HOW MANY ARE THERE?

There are 12 main meridians. An acupuncturist contacts these directly with a needle. Branching from them is a network of other smaller channels. The smallest channels are called 'cutaneous' meridians, and lie just beneath the skin.

Each meridian is connected to one of the twelve organs mentioned in the previous chapter. We'll look at two of these – the Gall Bladder and the Heart.

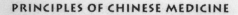

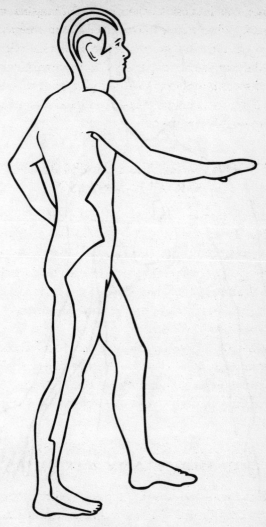

Gall Bladder Meridian

The Gall Bladder meridian begins beside the eye, travels around the side of the head then down the side of the body and the leg to end by the nail of the fourth toe (see picture). Many

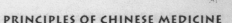

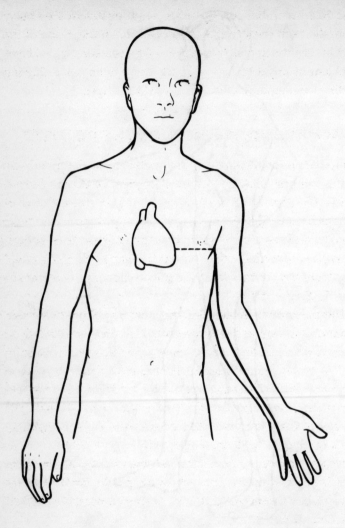

Heart Meridian

people have headaches travelling around this pathway at the sides of their heads and going to the eye. A needle in a point on the foot of this meridian often alleviates this type of headache.

The Heart meridian, on the other hand, trave[...]
from the heart itself to the armpit and down th[...]
arm to the little finger. This explains why someone[...]
problem or about to have a heart attack often has [...]
feeling running down the arm to the little finger.

WHAT ARE ACUPUNCTURE POINTS?

Acupuncture points lie along the pathways of the meridians. Points are best imagined as small vortices of energy formed where the flow of Qi is disrupted. They are often found at prominences or indentations along the pathways such as where a bone flares at a joint, where there is a notch in a bone or even where two muscles meet. This is similar to the way small whirlpools are formed when the smooth flowing of a stream or river is disrupted.

There are approximately 365 acupuncture points on the main channels, as well as many others which are not situated on main pathways. The Chinese sometimes discover a new point which proves extremely useful. For example, there is a point on the line of the Stomach meridian of the leg which becomes tender on pressure if a patient's appendix is inflamed. Think of the difference this could make to a doctor unsure about the diagnosis of a patient with abdominal pain!

Many acupuncture points can become tender with pressure. This is not always the case, however, and the point locations have all been specified so that an acupuncturist can find their exact locations.

CAN THE MERIDIANS BE SEEN OR FELT?

The meridians can rarely be seen by the human eye. They can, however, be felt. Often people practising qigong over a period

...ne (see chapter 6) become more sensitive to their Qi and are able to feel their pathways. Some people believe that this is how the pathways were originally found and traced out.

Patients often feel this energy travelling along their meridians close to where the needle is inserted. This may feel like a slight tingling sensation or even a numbness. One patient described what she felt when a point was treated, 'Whenever I had one particular point on my wrist treated I would feel a whoosh of energy travelling straight up the inside of my arm over my head and down my other arm. I then felt completely at peace and didn't want to move.' She had experienced the energy of her 'Heart' meridian moving through her meridian pathways. This created a feeling of well-being and relaxation.

Now that we have described what the meridians and points are, we'll look more closely at acupuncture treatment itself.

WHAT CAN ACUPUNCTURE TREAT?

It is important to bear in mind that an acupuncturist will diagnose in a holistic way rather than looking at individual symptoms. A practitioner diagnoses patients by evaluating their overall balance of Qi and does not use Western disease categories. It may be more appropriate to ask, 'Can this particular patient be helped by acupuncture treatment?' rather than 'Which diseases can acupuncture treat?'

An acupuncturist considers both mental and physical symptoms. The body and mind are linked and one area will affect another. For example, a female patient aged 37 had digestive problems which took root at a time of great unresolved anger and frustration. Acupuncture treatment smoothed the anger and at the same time resolved the digestive problem. She remarked, 'I began to feel more in control of my life and I no longer suffered from a churning stomach as I no longer felt "put upon" by other people like I had done.' Another patient, a man aged 54, had become very depressed after long years of chronic joint pains. As his physical problem eased and he became more mobile, he also began to feel better inside and his spirits naturally lifted. One of the first comments he made as he

Acupuncture treats these general areas of complaint

The following is a list of the general kinds of problems causing patients to come for treatment. They may have illnesses that include:

Breathing and lung problems such as asthma; chronic breathlessness; bronchitis; coughs; hayfever.

Circulatory problems such as angina; chronic heart conditions; high or low blood pressure; palpitations; poor circulation; stroke; thrombosis; varicose veins.

Digestive and bowel complaints such as inflamed gall bladder; gall stones; gastritis; indigestion; nausea; stomach ulcers; vomiting; colitis; constipation; diarrhoea; dysentery; irritable bowel syndromes.

Ear, eye, nose, mouth and throat disorders such as blurred vision; chronic catarrh; conjunctivitis; deafness; dry eyes; gum problems; nosebleeds; otitis media; sinusitis; sore throats; tinnitus; tonsillitis; toothaches.

Emotional and mental conditions such as anxiety; depression; eating disorders; insomnia; panic attacks.

Gynaecological disorders such as heavy periods; hot flushes and other menopausal problems; irregular periods; morning sickness; period pain; premenstrual tension; scanty or no periods; post-natal depression; vaginal discharge.

Joint problems and pain such as back problems; joint injuries or inflammations; headaches; osteoarthritis, rheumatoid arthritis, rheumatism; sciatica; Stills disease.

Neurological problems such as Bell's palsy; epilepsy; multiple sclerosis; neuralgia.

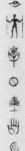

Sudden acute disorders such as the common cold; food poisoning; stomach upsets; influenza; mumps.

Skin conditions such as acne; eczema; psoriasis; urticaria.

Urinary and reproductive problems such as bedwetting; cystitis; impotence; urine retention; incontinence; infertility; kidney stones; prostate conditions.

became better was, 'I feel much better in myself.'

The list of problems mentioned in the box is by no means complete. It would be impossible to include all of the illnesses that acupuncture can treat and besides this there may not be a Western medical label for every problem. A patient may feel 'out of sorts' or 'lethargic and run down' or even 'not right but I don't know why'. Generally the acupuncturist's holistic approach is of great help in these situations and she will objectively advise the patient whether treatment is appropriate or not. To decide exactly what has caused specific problems and which treatment is needed, a thorough diagnosis is made. The patient is then ready for treatment.

WHAT IS IT LIKE BEING TREATED?

The patient usually lies on a treatment couch. The practitioner may first chat for a while to find out how the patient has been since the last treatment. She will then feel the patient's pulses and observe the tongue before inserting the needles into carefully chosen points.

The number of needles used depends on how acute or chronic the illness is and on the age, build and sensitivity of the patient. Usually anything from two to eight acupuncture points are used. The needles are either removed immediately after being inserted or sometimes they are left in place for 15 to 20 minutes while the patient relaxes on the couch. The time that the needles are left in varies according to the effect required on the patient's Qi.

Sometimes patients react to treatment even whilst lying on the treatment couch, for instance, one patient said, 'I always felt a change during the treatment. I was immediately better. It felt as if the energy is moving like a wave through my body, it was that strong.' Other patients don't feel any immediate change but feel the benefits later. For example, one 22-year-old builder commented, 'I didn't feel any different while the treatment was going on, but my backache soon felt better.'

HOW LONG WILL EACH TREATMENT TAKE?

A treatment will take anything from half an hour to an hour according to the practitioner and the needs of the patient.

JULIA'S WISHES COME TRUE

Julia is 35 and a teacher.

> 'I was desperate when I came to treatment. I wasn't getting anywhere with normal medicine. I'd had two miscarriages before I came and I wanted to conceive a baby naturally rather than take tablets. I needed someone to look at me as a whole person rather than as an illness.
>
> 'I was also easily upset and anxious. My mind would run away with me and I'd imagine all sorts of awful things happening to my husband. It got much worse before my period and sometimes even stopped me from sleeping well at night'.

Examination revealed that she was very hot, 'like a little radiator', however, her feet and lower abdomen always felt stone cold. The cold in the lower part of her body was making it difficult for her to conceive and remain pregnant.

Treatment was directed towards harmonizing her Kidney and Heart Qi, calming her spirit and warming her lower abdomen. After a few treatments she reported, 'I feel much less anxious and can stand back and see the imagined catastrophes for what they are'. During treatment her hands felt cooler and her lower body began to feel warmer. She reports:

> 'I was so desperate to sort myself out. Now I feel a hundred times better! Before, when I didn't feel well I couldn't handle anything. Things don't bother me now as they did. I feel much calmer and more peaceful inside. I'm more independent and I don't worry if my husband is out of the house. I'm physically and mentally on top and much more in charge of my life.'

Seven months ago she and her husband had some good news. She had become pregnant. They now eagerly await the birth of their baby.

HOW DOES THE THEORY OF CHINESE MEDICINE APPLY TO ACUPUNCTURE?

Most acupuncturists diagnose using the *Five Elements* and the *twelve organs* and will strive to find which organ is the root cause of a condition. Directing treatment towards this cause will rebalance the Qi of the whole person and restore health.

The acupuncturist is also concerned about the condition of the other *Substances* – the Blood, the Jing, the Body Fluids and the Mind-Spirit. The Substances can become deficient or obstructed in relation to an organ. The acupuncturist will fine-tune treatment directed towards that organ when she also knows which Substance is affected.

For example, an acupuncturist may realize that the patient's Liver is the underlying cause of the imbalance. A 35-year-old mother who came to treatment for scanty periods said, 'I have a slight tendency to get irritable after my periods but I never get very angry. I also get black spots in front of my eyes and often get muscle cramps.' Her skin was very dry. Her symptoms were caused by 'deficiency of the Blood of the Liver'.

A male patient aged 48 also had a Liver problem but his was caused by the Qi of his Liver not circulating properly and becoming 'stagnant'. He complained, 'I get severe migraine headaches which affect my eyes and I feel tired a lot of the time. I often feel angry and depressed and my mood changes very easily according to my situation at home or work.'

Both patients had a problem affecting the Liver but each manifested in a different way. This created a different emphasis on the points used for their individual treatments. Acupuncturists will also decide whether an External 'pathogen' is obstructing the energy balance in which case this needs to be cleared.

Treatment is carried out using needles and moxibustion as well as using other tools such as 'cups', a 'plum blossom needle' or a 'seven-star needle'. We'll now discuss all of these treatments starting with needles.

WHAT ARE THE NEEDLES LIKE?

The first needles that were used over 2,000 years ago were made from sharpened bamboo or from stone. Later on iron needles were used. Today, most acupuncture needles are made from stainless steel. This gives them certain important qualities. They are virtually impossible to break, they are very flexible and they will not rust. Gold and silver needles have also been used extensively and even now they are still used by a few practitioners.

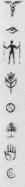

Acupuncture needles have a coiled handle and an extremely fine shaft with a sharp point. No substances are injected into

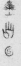

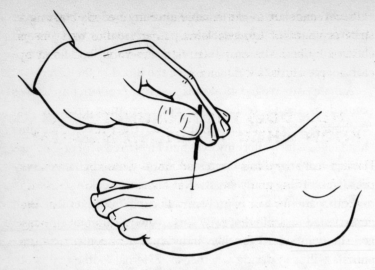

A needle being inserted

the body by the acupuncturist and therefore the needles are solid. In comparison, injection needles are thicker and hollow to allow medicines to be injected.

Acupuncture needles come in different lengths according to the area of the body which is to be treated.

HOW ARE THE NEEDLES STERILIZED?

Stainless steel needles are especially advantageous for an acupuncturist as they are easily sterilized. Most acupuncturists use single-use disposable needles which are made to a very high quality. Practitioners are happy to use disposable needles on any patient who requests them. Some acupuncturists have their needles sterilized in their local hospital autoclave, others have their own autoclave which they use on their premises. An autoclave cleans using 'steam under pressure' and is the most effective method of sterilizing needles or any equipment.

sign that there is more blockage of the Qi and a stronger needle manipulation has been required.

HOW IS MOXIBUSTION USED?

Needles and moxibustion are often used together in the same treatment. To create moxa the leaves of *artemesia vulgaris* go through a drying process until they resemble soggy cardboard! This is known as moxa 'punk'. Its appearance is somewhat deceiving. Anyone who has experienced moxibustion will confirm that it has a wonderful aroma and a powerfully warming effect. The distinctive aroma pervades most acupuncturists treatment rooms and is an important part of its use. As well as warming the Qi, the aroma of moxa is said to enter the meridians through the skin to stimulate the Qi and Blood.

Moxa can be shaped into small cones and placed on various acupuncture points to warm the body directly. It may also be used as a stick known as a moxa 'cigar'. When lit, this is held an inch or two from the skin and can warm anything from a small acupuncture point to a large area of the body. For deeper penetration of heat, moxa can be placed on the end of a needle and lit while the needle remains in the point. The warmth passes down the needle into the point and feels especially pleasant when a joint or particular part of the body is cold. Smouldering moxa placed in a specially made container called a 'moxa box' enhances this effect and can warm a large area of the body.

A 39-year-old radiographer describes her experience of moxa, 'It feels like a relief when I have moxa. I'm warmer inside and funnily enough I also feel warmer towards other people!' Another patient with a back problem says, 'I love the feeling of the moxa warming my back. I immediately feel less achy and more flexible there.'

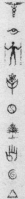

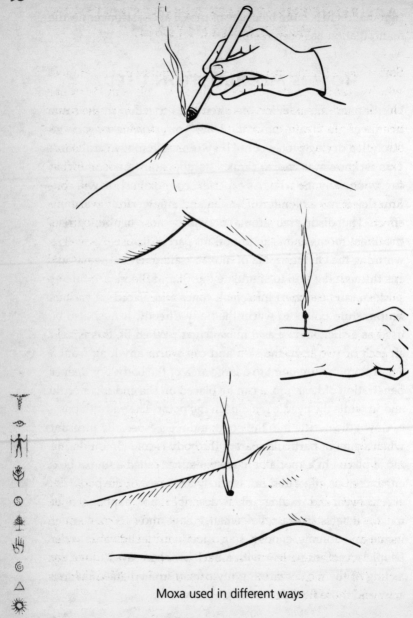

Moxa used in different ways

WHAT OTHER TREATMENTS MIGHT THE ACUPUNCTURIST USE BESIDES NEEDLES AND MOXIBUSTION?

Sometimes a practitioner may use a small lightweight 'hammer' which is tapped on the surface of the skin. This is made from a cluster of needles attached to a handle and is called a 'seven-star needle'. This 'hammer' can be used to clear blocked qi or to stimulate a specific area of the body. For instance, a patient had extremely painful and sore knees which made it difficult for her to climb stairs. She described them as stiff and aching. Her knees also looked very swollen. She benefited from the use of a seven-star needle around the knees as well as acupuncture and moxibustion to deal with the underlying cause of the problem.

A 'plum blossom needle' is similar to a seven-star needle and has been nicknamed a 'children's needle'. It can be used to tap points along the meridians on a child who does not wish to have needles.

Besides using needles and moxibustion an acupuncturist might also use 'cupping' to clear congestion.

WHAT IS CUPPING USED FOR AND HOW IS IT USED?

Cupping removes congestion in the body caused by obstruction by Wind, Cold or Damp (see Chapter 2).

Wind and Cold together can easily become lodged just under the surface of the skin especially around the upper back, causing the congestion associated with a cold and symptoms such as sneezing, a runny nose, achy joints and a slight headache. Many acupuncture points around the upper back have the word 'Wind' in their name and are used to clear Wind that has become 'stuck' in the body.

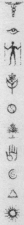

One way to clear a Wind-Cold is to suck it from the body using cups. A vacuum is created by placing a lighted taper into a glass or bamboo cup then quickly removing it before swiftly placing the cup onto the skin at the appropriate point. The cup is comfortably left in place for 10–15 minutes. After it has been removed the patient is told to wrap up warmly for a while as the Wind and Cold will be sweated out of the body.

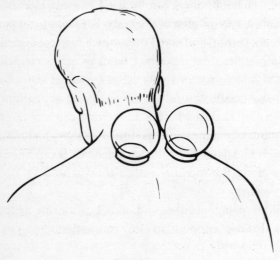

Cupping

Cupping on different areas of the body can also clear joint pains, backache or even some stomach upsets which have been caused by obstructions.

CAN I STILL HAVE ACUPUNCTURE IF I'M NOT ILL?

Yes, acupuncturists understand the importance of remaining healthy as well as being cured of specific illnesses. It is said that acupuncturists in China traditionally only charged their patients when they remained healthy. If they became sick the practitioner had been remiss in not foreseeing and preventing the condition and the patients stopped paying until their health was regained. This is one area where practitioners no longer follow the old traditions!

Many people come to treatment because they recognize the value of optimizing their health and energy even though they have no clearcut symptoms. Everyone can benefit from treatment and patients who are not ill often feel better and have more vitality, both immediately after being treated and in the longer term.

A 57-year-old headmistress describes what happened when she came for treatment:

> 'I'd heard about acupuncture and I felt alternative medicine was a good thing so I asked if I could have an "MOT". After the third treatment I'd had a horrendous day and still felt wonderful at the end of it and I realized that acupuncture had really made a difference. Work changed. Prioritizing became easy and instead of being at the back of a pile of work I was on top of things. Before, I had felt that I was rowing the boat underwater and against the current, now it's like rowing on top of the water and with the current.'

HOW WILL I FEEL AFTER A TREATMENT?

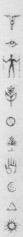

Reactions to treatment vary from person to person. Here are some observations made by patients after treatment: 'I always come out walking on air, it's like being smoothed out.' 'I love having treatment because I feel so much clearer and stronger inside afterwards.' 'Usually I don't experience a lot immediately after treatment but I have had some remarkable changes. Once I was in a heap just waiting to collapse. Within 5–6 minutes I felt very bright, not tired at all and totally alert.' 'I can't say I feel any change immediately. After the first treatment it was three days before I realized I hadn't taken a tablet.' Any of these reactions are considered to be a normal response to treatment. Rarely a patient may feel a slight worsening of symptoms for a short time before there is an improvement.

HOW MUCH TREATMENT WILL I NEED?

How long a person needs to come for treatment depends on how long she has been sick and the depth of the illness. As a general rule a patient can expect an acute condition such as severe back pain to be cured in just a few treatments while a long-term chronic one will take longer. An illness which started in childhood will often need many more treatments than one which started in adulthood. A severe and complicated condition such as a bowel problem with much bleeding and loose stools may need more treatments than a simple stomach upset.

A patient with a chronic condition usually starts coming to treatment once a week. As she improves, treatment will be spread out to once a fortnight, then monthly. In time the patient may be attending treatment only for a 'check up' at each change of season. Seasonal treatment helps to retain the balance of energy that has been achieved.

Sometimes the practitioner will propose that the patient makes dietary or lifestyle changes – such as cutting out fatty foods or getting more rest and relaxation. If these are issues that are affecting the patient's health she will considerably shorten her need for treatment by carrying out these suggestions.

AMY WALKS AGAIN WITHOUT PAIN

Amy's left knee swelled up and became sore when she went camping in damp weather twelve years ago. She is now 65 years old and has retired from her job doing accounts. The doctor told her she had arthritis and gave her painkillers which she didn't like taking. Four years later the right knee also started to swell up and feel painful. When she came for treatment a year later she told me, 'Some days I can't walk, I have to go up and down stairs on my bottom, my knees are so painful. The pain also keeps me awake at night.'

Upon examination her knees were found to be very swollen and stiff. They also felt cold to the touch and she confirmed that heat on her knees gave her some relief. Her diagnosis was an 'invasion of Cold and Damp' in her knees. This was exacerbated by an underlying Kidney and Spleen deficiency. Her knees were treated directly with moxa and needles and at the same time the underlying Kidney and Spleen deficiency was tonified as well.

After the first treatment she said, 'I feel great. Much better in spirits and my knees also feel better.' Now she reports on how life has changed.

'My life changed immediately. Two big warts I'd had all my life on my hand disappeared and I stopped having headaches. I began to feel fitter and fitter. The swelling in my knees soon went and I could walk without undue pain. The acupuncture worked with everything. I'd really thought that I'd be in a wheelchair within six months. My mother had been crippled with arthritis and I thought I'd go the same way. When I go to hospital for checks every doctor who has ever examined me says that they can't believe how well I am for my age and that my body is in perfect order. When I say I have acupuncture, they say it's obviously the right treatment for me.'

HOW DOES THE PRACTITIONER KNOW TREATMENT HAS WORKED?

A patient's immediate positive reaction to treatment is one sign that the treatment has been effective. There are many others that an acupuncturist can also observe. Most practitioners will feel the patient's pulses before and after treatment. An improvement in the quality of the pulses gives a reliable indi-

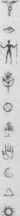

cation that treatment has been beneficial. Small changes in facial colour, voice tone or emotional state also signify a positive effect, or a new sparkle in the eyes shows that the spirit has lifted. Sometimes it is not obvious that treatment has worked until the patient returns to the next treatment and reports a change.

Before finishing this chapter we will look at two unusual ways of using acupuncture – acupuncture anaesthesia and ear acupuncture. Both of these have had much publicity in spite of being only a small part of the vast field of Chinese medicine. They can be useful treatments to use in certain situations.

CAN I HAVE ACUPUNCTURE ANAESTHESIA DURING AN OPERATION?

Acupuncture anaesthesia or analgesia (pain relief) is a relatively new area of treatment and was first discovered by the Chinese in the 1950s. They found that if certain acupuncture points on the body were stimulated, this would kill pain in specific areas. It has been used extensively for this purpose during operations carried out in Chinese hospitals.

Anaesthesia is especially beneficial for patients with problems in the upper area of the body and has been used in the West by dentists for tooth extractions. It can also be helpful to minimize pain during childbirth. One of its values is that few post-operative complications are created from its use so it could be helpful for sick or frail patients to whom it is too dangerous to give anaesthesia with drugs. Another is that a patient can remain conscious throughout treatment, although some patients would prefer to be put to sleep and wake up when it is all over!

Having said this, acupuncture anaesthesia is not yet readily available in the West. The majority of qualified acupuncturists work in their own private practices treating health problems and most have not specialized in this treatment. Anaethesia could be valuable for patients coming to a doctor's or dentist's surgery or a hospital where an acupuncturist was in practice. More opportunities are now available for cooperation between acupuncturists and doctors so there may be more of this treatment available in the future.

WHAT IS EAR ACUPUNCTURE?

Some acupuncturists use ear acupuncture in their practices, others do not. Ear acupuncture, like acupuncture anaesthesia, is relatively new and as yet forms only a small part of the spectrum of treatments in Chinese medicine. It is unclear whether this form of acupuncture was first discovered in the 1950s in France by Paul Nogier, or around the same time by the Chinese. Both developed this fascinating use of acupuncture simultaneously and made similar discoveries.

They found that there are points on the ear which coincide with every part of the body. These points correspond to a picture of a foetus with its head at the ear lobe, its internal organs in the deeper part of the ear called the conchae and its upper and lower limbs on the antihelix and the crura of the ear. This can be compared to reflexology where areas on the soles of the feet correspond with the different organs of the body and become sensitive to pressure when a person falls ill.

By examining the ear visually and probing for sensitive areas, a diagnosis is made and points selected for treatment. About 3–5 points are usually used. These may be treated using small acupuncture needles. Alternatively tiny seeds or ball bearings can be attached to the chosen spots using plasters. The seeds or ball bearings will stay in place on the ear for 3–4 days and can be pressed to stimulate the points.

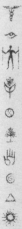

Ear acupuncture is useful for both acute and chronic problems and as an adjunct to other acupuncture treatment. It can be used for painful conditions and infections and may be effective for treatment during childbirth. It has been used extensively and successfully for withdrawal from drug dependency. A fellow practitioner who works with drug dependent patients in a London clinic frequently uses five special 'detox' points which are beneficial to stop craving for drugs. She also uses broader acupuncture treatment alongside the ear points to attend to other underlying conditions. By doing this she treats both the physical and psychological needs of her patients so that they can remain off drugs in the future.

Acupuncture is fast becoming a highly respected form of treatment. No other medicine has become so widely accepted in such a short space of time. Those who are put off by the idea of having needles inserted, quickly become converted once they start having treatment.

As one patient commented:

> 'I enjoy going for acupuncture treatment so much. I had imagined that I'd dread going – like when I go to the dentist, but it's not a bit like that. I look forward to going, I feel better while I'm there and I'm gaining huge health benefits physically and mentally as a result'.

Many of you could have these benefits too. All you need to do is pluck up the courage and try it – it'll be worthwhile.

CHINESE HERBAL MEDICINE
REMEDIES FOR YOUR ENERGY

C hristine was desperate when she first visited a Chinese herbalist. She had had period pains over a span of 8 years.

'They were in my lower abdomen and felt like knives sticking into me. The pain then continued for two weeks after the period and I felt as if I had been punched in the stomach. Before the period began my breasts swelled up and I often felt really angry and easily upset. It was ruining my life.'

The pain had started when she had a fallopian tube infection at the age of 23. The doctor had told her she had a disease called 'endometriosis' caused by small amounts of the womb lining breaking away and growing in other areas of the pelvic cavity. During menstruation this tissue caused her extreme pain.

The herbalist was sympathetic and prescribed herbs to move the Qi and Blood which she diagnosed as causing an obstruction in her lower abdomen. Christine boiled up the herbs and drank them daily. At the next period she was surprised to have no problem at all, 'I only had very slight and manageable pain.' After another month she had no more symptoms at all, the mood changes and the pain had all disappeared. 'It was a miracle!', she said.

She had been planning to move abroad for some time and when she finally left England her herbalist gave her some pills to take with her. These were to ensure that the symptoms did not recur. Six months later she wrote to say that the pain had never returned and that she had no more premenstrual problems. Not only that, she was extremely happy and contented with her new life.

Lindsey, aged 29 years and a university lecturer, had a different problem entirely.

'I felt foggy and woolly in my head and I had very little energy. I couldn't concentrate and was very depressed. Any energy I had to put into doing things would disappear. I was quite a mess. It felt like spinning plates waiting to crash!'

Lindsey was prescribed herbs to strengthen her 'Heart and Kidney' energy.

'I'd felt ill for about 4 years. After starting the herbs, in a matter of weeks I began to feel better. I now feel positive, my head is clear and I have good energy and concentration. I'm also much more consistent in how I feel. Before taking herbs I didn't know how I'd feel from one day to the next.'

These are just two examples of some of the spectacular results achieved by taking Chinese herbs.

Chinese herbs are very effective in the treatment of many medical conditions. Although they have been slower to grow in popularity in England than acupuncture, more and more people are now turning to these medicines as they hear about their beneficial effects.

In the rest of this chapter we will be looking at many aspects of Chinese herbal medicine. These will include how Chinese herbs differ from Western herbs, how a herbal prescription is prepared, what the different categories of herbs are and how they are used, as well as what it will be like to have treatment using Chinese herbal medicines and what kinds of conditions herbs can treat. Let's start by finding out more about Chinese herbal medicine itself.

WHAT IS CHINESE HERBAL MEDICINE?

The term 'Chinese herbal medicine' describes formulae which are made from the roots, stems, bark, leaves, seeds or flowers of many plants both wild and cultivated as well as some mineral and animal products. They are taken by over one billion people throughout the Orient and have been used for thousands of years. There are over 400 herbs in common use today.

The herbs are carefully prepared in a variety of different ways. They are frequently ingested in the form of dried herbs which are decocted into a soup, or as pills, powders or tinctures. Some external preparations are also used on the skin as ointments, creams or herbal plasters.

The herbal medicines are usually taken in the form of a 'recipe' known as a prescription. To make up a prescription the herbalist carefully blends together a number of herbs which have specific applications. Some of these herbs are so commonly combined together that they can be bought as a ready-prepared pill or powder. They are called 'patent' herbal remedies.

Many of the prescriptions being used today date back to around 200 BC when a famous herbalist called Zhang Zhong Jing wrote a book on how to deal with numerous common infectious diseases. He was the first person to systematize the use of herbs and the tradition continues to this day. Later in the chapter we'll look more closely at what is meant by a herbal prescription. First we'll evaluate the main distinctions between Chinese herbal medicine and Western herbs.

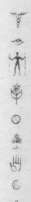

HOW DOES CHINESE HERBAL MEDICINE DIFFER FROM WESTERN HERBS?

There are two main differences between Chinese and Western herbal medicine. First, a Chinese herbalist diagnoses her patient using the theory of Chinese medicine. This is the same theory that is used by practitioners in all of the Chinese traditions mentioned in this book.

A Western trained herbalist will use a Western diagnosis which is the same as that used by Western doctors. This was not the original method of diagnosis used by herbalists in the West. Western herbal medicine, like its Chinese counterpart, has a long history. Unfortunately, much knowledge of this tradition has now been lost and this includes many of the diagnostic techniques. The understanding of many of the functions of the herbs has survived, however, and remains useful.

Secondly, the herbs are prescribed differently. A practitioner of Chinese herbal medicine will use a prescription made up of a combination of a number of herbs. These herbs will be chosen to fit the patient's energetic state. A Western herbalist prescribes herbs separately and will use individual herbs to treat a patient's complaint. Although a number of different herbs might be used, they will not be combined together into a prescription in the same way as Chinese herbs. Let's look in more detail at how the herbs are categorized and what we mean by a herbal prescription.

HOW ARE THE HERBS CATEGORIZED?

Herbs are categorized according to their main action and include herbs to 'Move Qi', 'Drain Damp', 'Scatter Cold' or 'Move Food Stagnation'. Tonic herbs which 'Tonify Qi' or 'Tonify Blood' strengthen the body when there is deficiency. Sadly there are very few 'tonics' found in Western medicine nowadays, although in the past they were often taken when a person felt 'run down' or 'out of sorts'. Today there are many people who feel depleted in energy and Chinese medicines can help to replenish exhausted energy.

Herbs can also be used to 'Calm the Spirit' when a patient is anxious or jumpy or to 'release the exterior' when a patient has an infection. Altogether there are more than 21 main categories of herbs that are blended together to make up a herbal prescription.

WHAT IS MEANT BY A HERBAL PRESCRIPTION?

There can be any number of ingredients ranging from one to twenty in a herbal prescription although six to eight is more usual.

The herbs are carefully balanced together. Prescriptions are constructed using a clear organizing principle in order to have the optimum effect on the patient. There are four main components in a prescription. These are the 'Emperor' herb, the 'Minister' herb, the Assistant or 'Adjutant' herb and the 'Messenger' herb. The component herbs have traditionally been named after different positions of responsibility in Chinese society. We will briefly discuss each of these components in turn.

The *Emperor* herb is the main herb in a prescription and may also be referred to as the *Sovereign* herb. Many people who have read the book or seen the film *The Last Emperor* understand the importance of the emperor in Chinese society. He was considered to be almost godlike in his position and carried out ceremonies and rituals which ensured the well-being of all of his subjects. The importance of this herb cannot be underestimated. This herb treats the main cause of the patient's imbalance and forms the highest proportion in the prescription.

The *Minister* herb has the job of assisting the Emperor herb or of treating another co-existing imbalance. Its job is similar to an important minister in the emperor's court. There is often more than one minister herb in a prescription and there is less of this herb in a prescription than of the Emperor herb.

The word *Adjutant* describes an army officer who does administrative work. This herb is added to the prescription to moderate any effects of the main herbs if necessary – the important administrative details we might say! For example, if the main herb is very tonifying to the Qi, the Adjutant herb may be added to move the energy so that it doesn't build up in one place but can also move around the rest of the body.

Finally, the *Messenger* herb. This has the job of carrying the other herbs in the prescription to the affected area and also of harmonizing all of the ingredients. The job of a messenger in the emperor's court was a lowly one but as essential as the position of the emperor himself. If the messenger stopped working the court would no longer run smoothly and harmonious relations among the subjects would break down. Traditionally, the Adjutant and the Messenger herbs make up the smallest proportion of the prescription.

HOW DOES THE HERBALIST CREATE A PRESCRIPTION?

Many prescriptions have been created by eminent herbalists over the last 2,000 years. These combinations are written about in Chinese herbal books and most of them have now been translated into English. Having diagnosed the patient's imbalance the herbalist can then choose which prescription is best suited to the patient and how it can then be modified to precisely fit her needs.

The practitioner will then add extra herbs, powders or

tinctures or subtract any unnecessary ones from the prescription. She may also change the quantities of the herbs being used. Finally the exact combination of ingredients are blended together to match the patient's requirements. If pills are used one or more of the 'patent remedies' can be combined.

HOW ARE THE HERBS PREPARED?

Most Chinese herbs used in the West are imported from China or Hong Kong. The herbs are all picked at the most appropriate time and prepared in advance.

Choosing when to pick each individual herb can be very important. Often the plants are picked when they are fully matured. The gatherer knows exactly which is the best time to harvest each herb. Many roots are most powerful in late autumn and early spring, whilst leaves are collected just before the flower reaches full bloom. The flower is then gathered later either in bud or in full blossom. Some fruits are used before they are ripe and need to be picked earlier; for example immature tangerine peel has a different effect to mature tangerine peel. Both move the Qi but the mature peel is used more in conditions relating to the Stomach and Spleen, whilst the immature one is often included in prescriptions for Liver complaints.

Once collected, the herbs need to be prepared. After being thoroughly washed and separated out, they are then usually dried in the sun or in a dry, well ventilated area. When they are thoroughly dry they are cut to a usable size, labelled and stored ready for use. The dried herbs can then be used to make herbal decoctions or they are made into pills, tinctures or powders.

WHAT IS THE DIFFERENCE BETWEEN DRIED HERBS, PILLS, TINCTURES AND POWDERS?

The most common way in which the herbs are used is in the form of a *herbal decoction* boiled up from dried herbs. The advantage of this method is that the herbalist can use the herbs in a fairly natural state and precisely weigh the quantities to be used. The herbs are then put into bags and are boiled up freshly every day. The disadvantage of using the dried herbs is that patients do not always want to boil herbs every day and must be highly motivated to do so.

Sometimes a herbalist will use *'patent' herbal pills* which have been prepared in China or the United States. Pills are made by grinding up the herbs then mixing them with honey or with another medium such as water or paste. They have the advantage of being easier to use than the dried herbs. Western people are more used to taking pills than to boiling herbs. The pills are often slightly cheaper than dried herbs and are commonly used for treating deficiencies or for acute problems. The disadvantages of pills is that the patent herbs don't cover every possible condition a patient may have and so they are not suitable in all circumstances.

Powders or tinctures are used slightly less frequently than decoctions or pills although they can be just as beneficial. *Powders* are ground up to make either a coarse or a fine powder. They can be taken directly or they are mixed with water and taken as a drink. Powders are now quite widely available from many distributors and are used as a matter of choice by some herbalists.

Tinctures are made by extracting the constituents of herbs in a mixture of alcohol and water. They are often taken by the spoonful or in water. Although tinctures are easy to take, their main disadvantage is that alcohol is known to have a slight heating affect on the body and so should be avoided in patients with hot conditions.

TWO USEFUL HERBAL PILLS FOR YOUR FIRST AID KIT

Two useful patent pills are 'Yunnan bai yao' and 'Yin qiao san'. Both are a must for the first aid cupboard.

Yunnan bai yao (pronounced You nan by yow) and translated 'Yunnan White medicine' is a must because it can literally save lives. The ingredients of this medicine are extremely effective and powerful and are carefully kept as a Chinese state secret!

This precious pill is used to cure any internal or external trauma. It will immediately stop shock, bleeding, pain and infection due to injuries, inflammation, post-operative trauma or internal problems such as intense period pains or heavy uterine bleeding. It can also be taken two days before operations to prevent post-operative shock. Many people can testify to its beneficial effects and I have known patients to undergo surgery with fewer post-operative problems than they could ever have expected.

It comes as a single red-coloured pill and about one eighth can be taken internally to heal wounds. In the case of serious injury the whole pill can be taken at once. This pill can also be crushed and applied to the outside of the body for external injuries.

The second useful pill for the first aid kit is *Yin qiao san* (pronounced Yin chow san) and translated 'honeysuckle and forsythia pills'. Yin qiao san can be taken at the first signs of a cold or when there is a sore throat or flu signs with a temperature, chills and muscle aches. Many of my patients take this to prevent colds from developing and often with great effect if the cold is caught in the early stages. There are two main herbs in this prescription and both are used to clear what is called

'Wind-Heat' from the system, hence it is especially beneficial if the infection is of a 'Hot' nature.

WHAT KINDS OF HERBS ARE USED IN A PRESCRIPTION?

Here is an example of a common herbal prescription and how it was modified to suit the needs of a patient. A 45-year-old man came for herbal treatment complaining, 'I need help with my digestive problems'. He had a very poor appetite and felt bloated and full after only a small amount of food. He also had slightly loose stools. When the practitioner enquired further he told her, 'My energy has been low for a long time. I also have difficulty concentrating and my head feels fuzzy and full up a lot of the time so that I can't think clearly.' His symptoms became worse in damp weather.

The herbalist diagnosed that his Spleen energy was deficient. One function of the Spleen according to the theory of Chinese medicine is to transform and move Fluids and Qi in the body. Because the Spleen was deficient the patient experienced a poor appetite and low energy. The Spleen energy was too deficient to move the body fluids and they were accumulating and causing him to have a bloated feeling and a muzzy head. The Chinese call this 'Internal Damp'.

The prescription that the herbal practitioner chose is one called 'The Four Gentlemen'. This prescription is made from a basic recipe containing four herbs. The *Emperor* herb in this prescription is 'ginseng', a herb that most people have heard of. Ginseng is a tonic and especially stimulates the Spleen energy. The *Mini-ster* herb is called 'white atractylodes'. Atractylodes also tonifies the Spleen as well as clearing some Damp and is used to assist the main herb. The third herb in the prescription is the *Adjutant* herb which is called 'poria'. Poria clears Damp in the Spleen and in this way modifies the action of the first two herbs so that they do not tonify the patient too strongly. Finally, the fourth *Messenger* herb in the prescription is 'baked licorice'. Licorice is a herb which blends together the other herbs in this prescription.

To modify the prescription to fit this patient more exactly the herbalist added two more herbs. The first one was 'tangerine peel'. This herb has a slightly stronger action of moving Damp. The second extra herb was 'pinella', which also dries up Damp as well as keeping the digestive organs warmed. The addition of these two herbs turns the prescription called the 'four gentlemen' into one called the 'six gentlemen'. The six gentlemen prescription will tonify the Qi of the Spleen and clear Damp.

On taking this prescription for some weeks the patient's symptoms cleared rapidly. He was delighted to find that his appetite improved, he stopped bloating after eating and he felt clearer in his head. He also said, 'I no longer fall asleep after my midday meal. It is a surprise as I'd thought it was a normal thing to do. In general I feel much stronger and have more energy.'

HOW IS THE THEORY OF CHINESE MEDICINE USED WHEN A HERBALIST DIAGNOSES A PATIENT?

When a patient goes for Chinese herbal treatment, the practitioner will carry out a diagnosis in much the same way as an acupuncturist. The aim of the diagnosis is to find out which of the 12 main *organs* are out of balance, how the *Yin and Yang* energies are balanced in relation to each other, which of the *Vital Substances* are deficient or obstructed and whether there are any *Pathogenic Factors* which need to be cleared from the body.

For example, a patient with eczema may be diagnosed as having an imbalance in one of the organs and a related

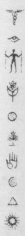

substance. Eczema can have many different causes and the herbalist will treat each individual differently according to the underlying root of the problem.

She may choose to treat the Qi of the Lung which is commonly associated with disorders of the skin or nourish the Blood of the Liver. The Liver Blood would normally moisturize the outside of the body. If it is deficient the skin can become dry.

The underlying Organ and Substance imbalance may cause the skin to be more easily 'invaded' by a pathogen from the outside. If the pathogen Wind-Heat invades the skin it creates a rash with a sudden onset that is hot, red, raised, painful and sometimes itchy. If Damp is involved the rash may ooze more or even become inflamed and pussy.

Imbalances are often caused by mental or emotional stress. Other causes may include a bad diet or exhaustion due to overwork.

Gathering information about the patient's problem is important for the practitioner to make a clear diagnosis. The diagnosis is made at the patient's first visit to the herbalist and in turn leads to precise treatment. The amount of time spent on the diagnosis depends on the individual patient and the practitioner and may vary from an hour to one and a half hours. Subsequent treatments take less time, usually from twenty minutes to three quarters of an hour.

After the diagnosis the herbalist will give the patient a prescription to send off to a herbal supplier. Some herbalists stock the herbs and will give them to the patients before they leave. The patient will also be given an appointment to return for the next consultation.

Six years ago Sally had glandular fever from which she didn't fully recover. She was later diagnosed as having 'myalgic encephalomyelitis', commonly known as 'ME', a post-viral syndrome. She is 46 years old, a trained doctor and is married with two children. She has been taking Chinese herbs for 18 months.

> 'I felt dried out and there was nothing left of my energy. I had terrible fatigue and exhaustion that went right to my bones, but even when I was lying down I still couldn't rest. I also had a tight chest, and was short of breath as if I was breathing in my throat. My digestion was terrible and I had nausea and very loose bowels. I'd have to run to the loo in the morning and afterwards I felt completely exhausted. I also had a permanent ringing sound in my ears, my back felt weak all the time and if I tried to walk anywhere my muscles would ache.
>
> 'I had mental symptoms that were even worse. I felt as if I had inflammation in my brain and I couldn't think straight, concentrate or take in information. I was in complete despair. It was as if my whole body was collapsing. I'd wake at night with night fears and a sense of total hopelessness and I'd have panic attacks during the day. I had thought my life was over and I was going to die and I was even suicidal at times. Taking the herbs was the turning point. As soon as I started taking them I knew I was going to recover.'

The first herbs were to clear the pathogen that had remained in Sally's system since the glandular fever. 'I felt different the next day. The terrible exhaustion began to lift and lighten.' After about a week she was given a herbal tonic and again felt dramatically different. 'I've got stronger and stronger ever since.'

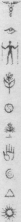

> 'Now all my physical symptoms have gone. I get mild ringing in my ears sometimes and a slight ache in my lower back. My digestion is better and I have no shortness of breath. My hair has started to grow back. Best of all I can now read books again and take in information. I can even dig my allotment without collapsing! I have a lot more energy and at times it feels normal. It's such a relief to feel better. I can look to the future now and it looks bright'.

WHAT CONDITIONS ARE COMMONLY TREATED BY HERBS?

All problems that can be treated by acupuncture can also be treated by a Chinese herbalist. Herbal medicines are used to treat many physical, mental, and emotional problems. Herbs have come to be known in the West as being especially beneficial for patients with skin conditions and gynaecological problems. They are also useful as tonics when patients have deficient Qi and Blood or for acute illnesses.

These are by no means all of the diseases that herbs can help. For a more detailed list of the general areas of complaints that herbs can treat, please refer to the list in chapter 4 on acupuncture.

WHAT DO THE HERBS TASTE LIKE?

The herbal decoctions or powders vary in their taste according to why they are being used. Pills are less variable in their taste than decoctions. They can be chewed or they can also be swallowed whole with water.

Here are some comments patients have made about the taste of herbs: 'I didn't mind the taste of herbs. When I didn't feel so well they were more difficult to get down.' 'I don't mind taking them. They are easy to take.' 'I boiled up the herbs my herbalist gave me. The taste was quite bland and I didn't mind drinking them.' 'They are definitely an acquired taste but I got used to them.'

The herbs have different tastes depending on why they are prescribed. To help us to understand more about this, we'll look at the way the Chinese classify the five tastes.

WHAT ARE THE FIVE TASTES AND WHAT DO THEY DO?

By using herbs over thousands of years the Chinese found that there are five main categories of tastes. The five tastes are *Pungent*, *Sour*, *Sweet*, *Bitter* and *Salty*. There is also a Neutral or Bland taste which has no clear flavour. Herbs are classified as having one or a combination of more than one of these flavours. The tastes each have differing effects on the body. The Sour, Bitter and Salty herbs are more Yin in their effect, that is, they have a downward moving and internal effect. The Sweet, Pungent and Neutral herbs are more Yang, as they have a more outward moving and exterior effect. Let's talk about each of these tastes in turn.

Pungent herbs are sharp and acrid in their taste and include common foods and herbs such as garlic, ginger, chilli pepper, black pepper, peppermint, and cinnamon. The effect of the Pungent taste is to disperse and move obstructions in the Qi and Blood and should be taken with care by a patient with very deficient energy. They are often used when people have colds and flus and will clear an infection by opening the pores and promoting sweating. The sweating thus eliminates the pathogen that has caused the illness.

Sour herbs have the opposite effect to Pungent ones in that they stop discharges and are astringent in their action. They are used to help problems such as urinary incontinence, excess sweating, haemorrhaging or diarrhoea. Sour herbs and food which we can recognize include vinegar, unripened plums, lemons and crab apples.

The *Sweet* flavour described in Chinese medicine is a subtle flavour, different from the strong sugary taste of sweet that is often used in the West. It is probably one of the most frequent tastes found in food and herbs and includes common herbs

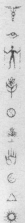

such as licorice, Chinese dates and ginseng as well as many vegetables, fruits and meats such as carrots, lamb or sweet potatoes. The sweet taste if taken in small quantities will have a tonifying effect on our bodies though in excess it will have a Dampening effect. *Bland* tasting herbs or food also have a slightly tonifying effect.

The *Bitter* taste cools and travels downwards through the body. It will remove Heat and clear the body and is used to stimulate the digestion, to cool fevers and to clear bowel problems due to heat. Because of its purging action on the body it, like the Pungent taste, should not be used in large quantities when a person has deficient energy. Some examples of common Bitter herbs and foods are rhubarb, dandelion, chicory and bitter oranges.

Finally, the *Salty* flavour is found in foods and herbs such as algae, seaweeds and seafoods like mussels, oysters and cuttle-fish. The salty taste will soften hard lumps in the body causing anything from a nodule below the skin to a goitre. This taste will also act as a diuretic and will clear excess water from the system.

This description of the five tastes and their effects demonstrates why some prescriptions taste different from others. A tonifying herbal prescription will taste more Sweet than a purging one which can be quite bitter. A prescription for an astringent will be more Sour tasting than a Pungent one which may be used to clear the system of an infection.

For a more complete list of food tastes see Chapter 8 on dietetics.

WHAT ARE THE FOUR ENERGIES AND HOW ARE THEY USED?

Along with the five tastes, the four energies are also important when deciding on the correct herbs for a prescription. The four energies are *Hot, Warm, Cool* and *Cold* temperatures. Most people in the West don't realize that knowing the temperatures of foods and herbs can be very useful when we choose what to eat in our diets. To the Chinese, the temperature of herbs or food is not decided by whether they are physically hot or cold but by the Heating or Cooling effect they have on the body. The temperatures of foods are described in more detail in chapter 8.

HOW OFTEN WILL I NEED TO VISIT MY HERBALIST AND FOR HOW LONG?

The Register of Chinese Herbal Medicine (RCHM) states that a practitioner must see a patient to check on her progress at least once a month. Most patients visit a herbalist for the treatment of long-term chronic problems. They will be seen by the practitioner for a new prescription every three to four weeks.

It is difficult to be precise about the length of time that is needed to cure any one patient as everyone is different. The length of treatment will depend on the patient's underlying constitution and strength of Qi as well as the condition being treated. Treatment will vary from weeks or months to over a year if the problem is more severe. Throughout the course of treatment the patient will be progressing towards a better balance of health.

If a patient has an acute problem such as a cold, cough, urinary or other infections or stomach or bowel upsets then herbs can also be very helpful. In the case of an acute condition the herbalist will want to see the patient more frequently and may prescribe herbs for a few days only. Treatment for acute conditions is less prolonged than for more chronic ones.

As with all of the Chinese therapies it is important that a Chinese Herbalist is well qualified. Membership of the Register of Chinese Herbal Medicine is one way of ensuring this. The Register of Chinese Herbal Medicine gives clear guidelines

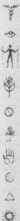

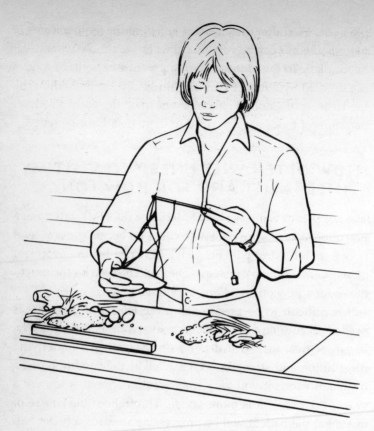

A traditional herbalist weighing herbs

which ensure the careful use of all herbs which are used in treatment.

MARGARET'S PSORIASIS IS MAGICKED AWAY

Margaret came to treatment with a skin condition called psoriasis when she was 64 years old. It had come on badly 2½ years before although she had always had allergic tendencies. 'There was a change in my home circumstances', she said matter-of-factly, 'my husband retired and things were very difficult to begin with.' She then went on to say:

> 'I tried every cream the doctors could prescribe, but I wanted to get to the inside of the problem rather than putting ointment on. It was practically all over my body, my legs, my arms, in my hair, even in my ears, my nails and the bottom of my feet. It covered 85 per cent of my body. The skin looked red and raised and it was very flaky. My legs were completely red and there was very little clear skin. My body was covered all over in red areas the size of a ten pence pieces.'

Margaret took Chinese herbs for about 3 months then suddenly and spectacularly her arms and body cleared overnight. 'I couldn't believe it!' she said.

Margaret still sounds surprised as she relates this story. A few patches on her elbows and a patch at the top of her left leg remain. Her nails and feet have cleared completely and her hair is almost clear. She looks forward to the time when she is completely cured of her symptoms but is delighted with the change so far.

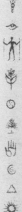

6

QIGONG EXERCISES
TRANSFORMING YOUR ENERGY

'I started learning qigong when I visited China three years ago,' a colleague told me recently. 'I was only there for four weeks and it wasn't long enough to learn many of the exercises in depth and yet I gained so much from doing them that I decided to find a teacher as soon as I returned to England. After I'd returned home I went to visit an acquaintance because she also practised qigong. I was surprised to find that the exercises she called qigong were completely different from those I had learned but the interesting thing was that she'd benefited just as much from her practice as I had from mine'.

What my colleague had discovered was that qigong (pronounced Chee gong) is an umbrella term that covers a vast array of Chinese exercises. The word 'qigong' was coined in China in the 1950s and covers sitting, standing and moving exercises all used for specific purposes. Many of these exercises had previously been closely guarded secrets which were passed down within families or from master to pupil over thousands of years.

Qigong practice mushroomed in popularity in China in the mid-1980s. Encouraged by increased freedom in China, many qigong masters came out of hiding and taught their craft to the people. Thousands of Chinese people rediscovered their heritage and learned the exercises to strengthen and transform their Qi energy. At one time it was said that one in five members of the Chinese population did some form of these 'internal' exercises.

Strange and exciting stories of qigong masters circulated – miraculous feats like turning on light bulbs with Qi energy, breaking rocks with the head or even affecting the weather. Some of the stories may have been true, others more in the realm of myth but they all added to the attraction and mystique of the exercises.

The excitement has died down now in China but many Chinese, young and old, are still seriously practising these exercises on a daily basis. Many of the qigong masters have come to the West attracted by serious students who, like my friend, want to find out more.

My colleague found that her colleague's teacher suited her. She now practises qigong on a regular basis at home and sometimes goes to classes to practise in a group. She says she feels much healthier and has more vitality as a result.

So what is the essence of this ancient and fascinating form of exercise that entranced so many Chinese and is now captivating Western people as well?

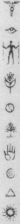

WHAT IS QIGONG?

The word 'qigong' (called Chi Kung in some books) is made up of two words 'Qi' and 'gong'. We have already examined the word 'Qi' in the first chapter of this book. It loosely means 'energy' and a little more precisely 'the force that underlies everything in the universe'. The word 'gong' can be translated as 'practice'. The word qigong conveys the meaning of 'practice concerned with Qi' or we might even say, 'any practice which is concerned with exercising our Qi'.

In the rest of this chapter we will be exploring this 'exercising of our Qi' and discovering how types of qigong differ as well as how they are similar. We'll consider the theory behind qigong, how it compares with exercises traditionally done in the West and how to practise it. We'll also look at some simple exercises and how qigong can benefit us.

WHAT ARE THE BENEFITS OF PRACTISING QIGONG?

Some of the reasons why people say they practise qigong are to improve health, for spiritual development and to keep healthy. Many practitioners of acupuncture or massage say they do qigong 'to improve my healing ability'. Qigong has also been used by those who practise martial arts as a way of increasing the power of their fighting techniques. We will not be covering this application in this book. Let's now look at the other benefits individually.

HOW COULD QIGONG IMPROVE OR MAINTAIN MY HEALTH?

Improving and maintaining health was one of the first uses of qigong and it is mentioned in *The Yellow Emperor's Classic of Internal Medicine* written in about 200 BC. Chinese doctors realized that gentle exercise can stimulate the flow of our Qi. We already know that when our Qi runs smoothly throughout our bodies we remain healthy. If our Qi is blocked or weakened this results in ill health.

There are many reasons why our Qi becomes obstructed or weak. One major cause of illness is tension or emotional upsets. These may cause us to tighten up inside and constrict the movement of our Qi. Short-term problems will resolve themselves fairly easily, but more long-term emotional problems will upset the healthy flow of our Qi.

The gentle qigong exercises stimulate the circulation of energy in the body to improve our health. Some of the exercises are specifically designed to improve the functioning of different organs in the body. For example, some exercises will help to improve the Kidney, Liver, Lung or Heart function, whilst others are aimed directly at other functions such as helping the digestive system, improving the circulation or clearing the head. Some exercises have been found to help people to lose weight. One exercise called 'the dragon swimming exercise' has been used extensively by people in China for this purpose. Most exercises have more than one beneficial effect. For example, the dragon swimming exercise also strengthens the Kidneys, the spine and the lower abdomen (see page 92).

Other exercises improve our health in a more general way by creating a better balance of Qi throughout our system. Maintaining this balance of Qi in the body is one of the best methods of health maintenance.

The practice of all of the exercises induces a calm and peaceful feeling and this in itself creates good health. Huang Fu Mi (pronounced Hwang Foo Mee) was a famous Chinese physician who was born in AD 215. He suggested that the best form of treatment is carried out *before* a disease has manifested. Qigong is one way in which we can stop disease from occurring as well as positively improving our health.

A 43-year-old translator who practises regularly says, 'One reason why I practised qigong is that it had an immediate impact on my health. I realized that qigong could make very quick improvements in things like headaches, indigestion and incipient colds and that has encouraged me to carry on.' Another woman, aged 44, who practises every day comments, 'I have lost weight, I eat less, I have more energy and I need less

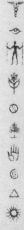

sleep. Emotionally I feel less stuck and my mind is freer.'

Whether Qi exercises are initially used for spiritual development or for better health, continued health maintenance is a positive side effect.

HOW DO PEOPLE USE QIGONG FOR SPIRITUAL DEVELOPMENT?

One 38-year-old teacher says of his qigong practice, 'As I practise I start to feel more harmonious and vibrant yet still, I also feel more aware and connected.' A 34-year-old woman from London said, 'I feel more integrated within myself and more in the moment. I have even had some insights into life and death.' These people and many others have become aware that practising qigong hasn't only had an effect on their health but it has also altered their consciousness of their connection to the universe.

Qigong exercises include many techniques for cultivating spiritual energy. One of the most well-known methods is called the 'small circulation of Qi'. To cultivate Qi, it is drawn up along a main energy pathway that travels up the back of the body called the 'Du' channel and then directed down a connected pathway at the front of the body called the 'Ren' channel. The energy is moved by using breathing exercises or concentrating on points along the two channels. The movement then starts to transform our Qi as it circles around the body and will in turn enhance our Shen or Mind-Spirit and our spirituality. Although many qigong exercises are rooted in Taoism and Buddhism, the practice of qigong for our spiritual development does not entail any religious commitments or observances.

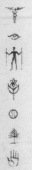

CAN QIGONG REALLY BE USED TO HEAL PEOPLE?

Yes. People usually begin to practise the different exercises to help maintain their own health. As their energy transforms, however, they may find that they can transmit and use the extra energy to heal others. This kind of Qi is called 'external Qi' and it is emitted because the 'internal Qi' has become strong and is flowing without obstruction. Many practitioners who use acupuncture, massage or healing like to develop this ability to use when they practise.

One acupuncturist mentioned recently, 'I find it necessary to practise qigong alongside practising acupuncture and find it enhances my results.' Another commented, 'Since I learned qigong my needle technique is more powerful and I am more sensitive to my patient's needs.'

A CURE FOR STEVE'S SHOULDERS

Steve's shoulders had been a problem for so long that he had resigned himself to them being achy and stiff nearly all the time. The problem had started fifteen years before when he had a job which strained his shoulder area. At the same time the break-up of a relationship put him under severe emotional strain. 'Sometimes they weren't too bad at all but if I'd been working hard or if the weather was damp they'd be much worse.'

He was 45 years old when he heard about a qigong course that was about to start, and was especially attracted when he heard about the health benefits qigong might bring. During the first few lessons he learned a number of different exercises aimed at strengthening his Qi. He was told that one particular exercise was especially helpful for the shoulders so he spent more time doing this. His teacher was well known for his healing ability and for projecting 'external Qi', so Steve also went to him for treatments.

> 'He sat me down and stood with his palms facing me and started moving his hands so that he projected Qi towards me. He was about one metre away from me and he didn't touch me. As he was making these movements I could feel his energy very powerfully. In fact it was so strong that I started to sway and found I couldn't resist the strength of it.'

Steve was surprised to find that his shoulders felt much better even after the first treatment. With a few more treatments and regular qigong practice he had no more trouble with them. That was three years ago.

> 'My shoulders have been much better ever since that time. I still regularly practise my qigong exercises because I enjoy doing them and because I feel much healthier now. I have more stamina and energy generally than I ever had before so I can't imagine a time when I'll want to stop.'

IS IT TRUE THAT PRACTISING QIGONG HELPS PEOPLE TO DEVELOP OTHER SPECIAL ABILITIES?

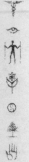

Although regular qigong practice can indeed help people to develop special 'gifts' such as seeing or hearing at a distance, knowing the future, or seeing a person's internal organs to read their state of health, this should be regarded merely as a bonus that results from much practice rather than as an expectation. Some qigong masters became famous for developing these special abilities but only gained them after much long practice. So don't expect to be reading other people's minds too quickly!

WHAT DO THE DIFFERENT QIGONG PRACTICES HAVE IN COMMON?

We emphasized earlier that qigong exercises are all different. However it's also important to note that they have many similarities.

First, they are usually performed very slowly and gently. Sometimes the only movement taking place is on the inside of the body and the person appears to be completely still on the outside. They can be broadly grouped into four main categories which are:

1 sitting exercises

2 standing exercises

3 moving exercises

4 spontaneous moving exercises

Secondly, whether there is external movement or not, the mind is usually kept focused during the exercises. The attention may be directed internally on a movement or a visualization or on an area in the lower abdomen called the *tan tien*. Sometimes the mind is projected outwards into the distance to increase the ability to transmit Qi, or in a healing situation someone with experience might direct Qi towards another person. This concentration develops 'mental power'.

Thirdly, although people practise qigong for various different reasons, all agree that one of the end results is to feel calmer and more relaxed. They also feel healthier and have a greater sense of well-being if they practise regularly.

Fourthly, one of the theories behind this practice is that we can unblock and strengthen the Qi energy that runs in the

meridian pathways (see chapter 4) and that the exercises are generally aimed at cultivating and transforming the energy. Let's now discuss more of the theory behind using these exercises and find out how much of it, if any, is needed in order to actually do qigong.

HOW DOES THE THEORY OF CHINESE MEDICINE FIT IN WITH QIGONG PRACTICE?

Anyone who decides to practise qigong may hear the words *Yin/Yang* and *Five Elements* mentioned fairly often. They may also notice the words, *Kidney, Liver, Heart, Spleen, Stomach* or *Lungs* being referred to more in a Chinese than a Western context. In spite of the frequent use of these Chinese medical terms, knowledge of Chinese medical theory is not necessary in order to do qigong.

The person who practises qigong does, however, need to learn how to do the exercises correctly as well as understanding why she is using them. If she then uses the exercises she will experience the beneficial effects.

When practising the exercises a person might notice tingling feelings, numbness, or a rushing feeling as the energy moves. Often these sensations will be found to correspond exactly to the pathways of the meridians which are referred to in more detail in chapter 4. As we mentioned earlier, one of the aims of some forms of qigong is to open up the pathways of the twelve main meridians as well as the 'Du' and 'Ren' channels on the back and front of the torso. When all of these channels are open and balanced the natural result is good health and a feeling of well-being.

In chapter 1 we examined the 'Vital Substances' which are the underlying matter from which we are made. In the practice of qigong, the *Jing* or essence, the *Qi* and the *Shen* or Mind-

Spirit are the most significant substances. Together they are known as the 'three treasures'. By exercising our Qi on a regular basis we can strengthen these three substances and increase our vitality and well-being.

The most important area of the body to be strengthened and activated is the *tan tien* which is situated in the lower abdomen and is the seat of our *Jing* or essence.

WHY IS IT IMPORTANT TO ACTIVATE THE TAN TIEN?

The Jing is the root of our constitution and vitality. By activating the *tan tien*, which is approximately four finger widths below the navel, the vital energy which is stored there is awakened. When this region starts to become active a vibration can sometimes be felt in the area and it may feel warmer. Awakening the energy in the tan tien conserves our supply of Jing and in turn strengthens our Qi. This is important for our overall health as well as for our spiritual development. As this energy builds it will also help to develop external Qi which can be used for healing.

HOW DO I ACTIVATE THE TAN TIEN?

There are three main ways to strengthen the *tan tien*. Breathing into this area is one way of developing it. Deep breathing into the lower abdomen naturally relaxes us and this in turn builds our energy.

Adjusting our posture during qigong exercises so that the centre of gravity naturally falls to the tan tien will also aid its activation. (See diagram of the basic standing posture.) A third way is merely by putting our attention on this area in the lower abdomen, a very simple yet effective way to strengthen it.

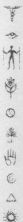

If we develop a strong internal centre we become strong, our energy becomes focused and our mind clear. Without this centre we will be weaker and more prone to ill health.

One 30-year-old mother of a three year old mentioned, 'Since I have been doing qigong I feel that my body can recentre itself almost spontaneously. I find it much easier to bring about a balance and clear my system and I often practise whilst walking or playing with my son.'

HOW ARE QIGONG EXERCISES DIFFERENT FROM EXERCISES USUALLY DONE IN THE WEST?

If we compare qigong exercises to those that are traditionally done in the West we will notice that the major difference is *what* is being exercised.

Exercises such as running, jumping, swimming, cycling or playing competitive sports all involve *exercising the physical body* only. This exercise is quite vigorous. The body grows stronger and fitter as a result, but changes to the mind and spirit are not emphasized. The Chinese call such exercise 'external' exercise as only the outside is being moved.

Qigong practice *exercises our Qi*. Our Qi is moved by directing our concentration to a specific area such as the tan tien described earlier. The movements of qigong tend to be gentler and more relaxed than purely physical movements. The result of qigong practice is that we become calmer and more serene inside as well as healthier physically as *both* the body and the mind are affected. Because Qi energy circulates on the inside of the body most qigong exercises are called 'internal' exercises.

The Chinese do not discount the beneficial effect of external exercise. In fact most Chinese people regularly do external exercise when they cycle to work. They do not, however, think that this is the only way of exercising. Both styles of practice are useful for different reasons.

WHAT ARE THE DIFFERENT TYPES OF QIGONG EXERCISES?

We mentioned earlier in the chapter that the main types of qigong are sitting, standing, moving and spontaneous moving qigong. We will look at them individually to get a better sense of what they are used for. Most qigong teachers will be experienced in teaching more than one of these different styles. First, 'sitting' qigong.

The term *sitting qigong* describes meditation exercises which are all aimed at cultivating the Qi for better health or spiritual development. The first stage of qigong meditation is often to sit and concentrate or breathe into the tan tien as was explained earlier when we described the process of activating the tan tien. The small circulation of energy up the back and down the front of the body is also a form of sitting qigong. Another useful meditation exercise is rotating the tan tien. This can be the first stage of awakening the tan tien.

ROTATING THE TAN TIEN

1 Sit upright on a chair with the knees and feet shoulder width apart.

2 Breathe in while pulling in the abdomen as much as possible towards the back and at the same time pull up the anus. This will create a force starting from the base of the spine going upwards to the middle of the back.

3 Continue to breathe in and pull up the anus so that the force continues to travels up each vertebra of the spine to the level of the waist. The force going upwards will open the back.

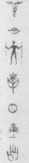

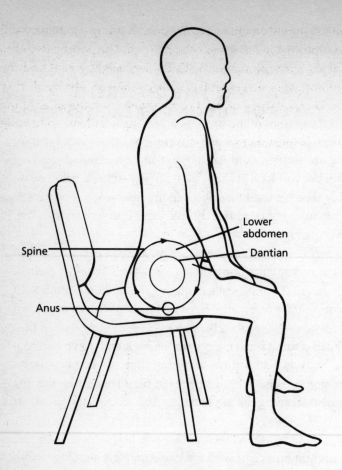

Circulating Qi in the lower abdomen

This opening will then make the force change direction and start to move forwards.

4 When you feel the direction changing, breathe out and relax the abdomen and anus. The force will then go downwards.

5 Repeat steps 1–5 for a few minutes. As a result a circular movement will occur in the tan tien.

Standing qigong describes exactly that, standing completely still in one posture in order to develop the Qi. The posture itself has to be correctly positioned with the legs slightly bent and the head upright so that the full benefit is achieved. The hands may be held in a variety of positions varying from the sides of the body, to in front of the body as if holding a balloon, to holding the hands together in a prayer position.

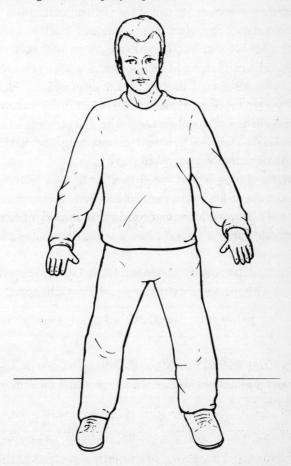

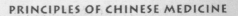

Basic standing posture

Standing still develops the concentration and mental power as well as facilitating the flow of Qi throughout the body and strengthening the tan tien. By standing in one place the legs are strengthened because energy is drawn up into the body from the earth.

There are many *moving qigong* exercises, some of which are well known and others which are less so. Some of the most well-known exercises are called the 'five animal frolics' which were developed by Hua Tuo, a famous doctor who lived between AD 120 and 208. These exercises are still very popular today and are performed in numerous different ways. The 'eight brocades' are another set of famous exercises which were developed in the Song dynasty (AD 1127–1279) by an army officer who wished to maintain the health and strength of his soldiers. These exercises are still maintaining the health and strength of numerous people to this day.

Moving qigong is performed in a gentle and relaxing way. The movements tend to be performed slowly although they can sometimes be done more vigorously. It is important to remain concentrated and in a good posture while doing them.

DRAGON SWIMMING EXERCISE

1 Stand with the feet together or shoulder width apart.

2 Hold the palms of the hands pushed tightly together with the fingertips pointing upwards.

3 Move from the tan tien. Move the hands in three circles going up and down the body to create a spiralling movement. (See also page 93.)

Finally, *spontaneous moving qigong* is perhaps the most unusual form of qigong. The qigong practitioner will stand in the position prescribed by the teacher and then relax. After a while

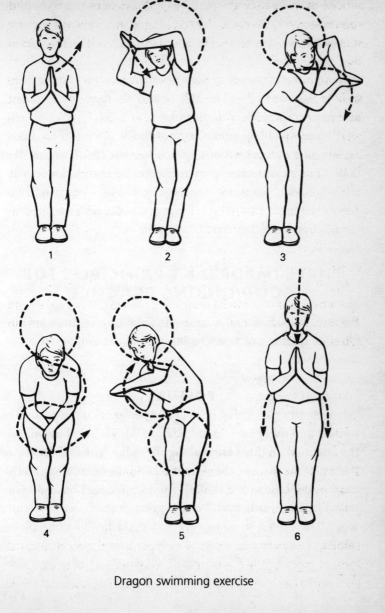

Dragon swimming exercise

small movements will start in the body. The person may shake, vibrate or move in other spontaneous ways or even make spontaneous sounds. As the Qi starts to move in the body it encounters blocks in our system. The spontaneous movement arises as our Qi pushes through these blockages and clears them. Although the person is moving spontaneously it is interesting to note that she will still be able to stop the movements at will and remain completely in control.

The purpose of spontaneous movement is to clear the body of any illness, obstructions or stuck emotions. Clearing the body of its sickness is important before the energy can be revitalized. Spontaneous moving qigong is often practised in a group setting at first where the movements are instigated by the teacher. Later they may be done alone.

THREE IMPORTANT PRINCIPLES FOR GOOD QIGONG PRACTICE

Posture, relaxation and a focused mind are the three keys to effective qigong practice. Qigong techniques emphasize all of these in some way.

POSTURE

When standing or sitting it is very important that the posture is upright and the spine remains straight. This is aided by putting the attention on three areas along the spine. The first area is at the top of the sacrum, the second behind the heart area and the third at the base of the skull. If they are focused on and mentally lifted upwards it will create good posture which in turn will allow the Qi to run freely and good health to be maintained.

Many people think they are relaxed if their body becomes limp. We wouldn't be able to practise qigong in a relaxed way if this were the case as we would be in a heap on the floor! The relaxation of qigong is very alive and dynamic because our mind is focused as we relax. This creates a 'living' relaxation rather than a 'dead' and floppy relaxation. This relaxation is important as it also helps to free the energy flow and enhance our vitality.

A FOCUSED MIND

A focused mind is the third string to the qigong bow. There is a saying that 'where the mind goes our energy follows' and this is certainly true when it comes to qigong practice. Whether we direct our mind inwards or outwards it needs to be fully involved in whatever exercise we are doing and at the same time remain relaxed and calm. To use internal visualization, for example, a person may imagine that she is standing holding a large ball between her hands. The ball may be kept still or be slowly moved upwards, downwards, from side to side or rotated backwards or forwards. The exercises are performed in a relaxed way and an upright posture is maintained. The addition of the imaginary ball adds the mental component to what would otherwise be undirected movement.

Combining good posture, a focused mind and relaxation when we exercise our Qi enhances the experience we have when practising qigong. This can result in improvement to our health and may mean that we finish our practice with an inner sense of well-being or an extra sparkle in our eyes.

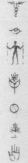

HOW WILL I FEEL WHILE PRACTISING QIGONG?

There are some generalizations that can be made concerning what happens during qigong practice but this will vary according to which exercise is being done and who is doing it.

Although some people have an immediate positive experience when they first start to practise, it can take plenty of motivation and much determination to continue to practise regularly and feel the beneficial effects. In fact some of the exercises can feel painful at first. The arms may be held in one position over a long period of time causing muscles to ache and new muscle groups may be used. Spontaneous moving qigong can appear very strange when you are new to qigong!

The effort is worth it. The later positive effects far outweigh the initial discomfort and all will be forgotten as the feelings of well-being manifest.

Here are some comments people have made about their experiences during qigong practice: 'I often get a sense of my Qi "shaking down" and beginning to flow more smoothly as well as a sense of warmth and general well-being.' 'It can vary enormously from very serene to quite disturbed, but it usually settles into a more harmonious feeling of being more aware and connected.' 'I sometimes feel "big" sensations – my hands can feel enormous, I feel movements in places where I usually don't move.' 'There is a definite change in my state of mind, it becomes quieter and I feel an expansion beyond my physical body, I feel like I fit into one of the slots in the universal puzzle.'

HOW CAROL BENEFITED FROM QIGONG

'Before I started practising qigong I was very depressed,' Carol told me. 'In fact it's hard to recognize me now because I feel so different.'

'I felt heavy and pessimistic about everything, but also very unsettled and nervous all the time to such an extent that I could never keep physically still. I only went to a qigong class because a friend was going and persuaded me to go along too – I decided that it would be better than sitting at home smoking cigarettes and feeling bad, but I wasn't very interested.

'From almost the first session I noticed something was different – I felt more expressive and outgoing, my voice had more volume and I noticed an inner feeling of peace. This gradually built up although at first I felt better after some classes than others.

'Now I can honestly say that qigong has transformed my life. I sleep better, I feel much calmer and I no longer move about like I used to, my head is clearer and I am a stronger, more positive person altogether. As well as doing formal qigong practice every day I also try to bring it into my work as a gardener. For example, when I'm doing things like raking leaves, digging or cutting hedges I find that I can do them in such a way that I feel energized instead of worn out as I would have done before.'

There are three added bonuses for Carol. One is that as she felt better she also found the strength to give up smoking. The second is that she met someone at the class and she now has a committed relationship with him and the third added bonus is that they practise qigong together.

HOW WILL I FEEL IMMEDIATELY AFTER PRACTISING QIGONG?

We have already looked at qigong's beneficial long-term effects, whether used for healing, health maintenance or spiritual development. Here are some observations people have made concerning how they feel immediately after practising. A 40-year-old mother of two says, 'I have an immediate feeling of relaxation yet alertness and "aliveness", a sense that anything is possible and that I'm no longer restrained by my own

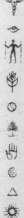

98   self-limitations'. Another comment was made by a 42-year-old Londoner, 'Troubles of the mind disappear! I feel cleansed, very centred and I usually feel happier.' The next comment by a 35-year-old computer programmer reflects a common experience, 'I feel increased calmness and more aware of what is going on around me.' Finally, a comment from a man of 45, 'I have more feelings of well-being, feel free of stress, exercised and energized and clearer mentally.'

DO I NEED TO HAVE A TEACHER?

The simple answer to this is yes. Exercises practised badly can be dangerous. Each qigong exercise is carried out in a specific way that requires feedback on posture and the technique of performing the exercise. In China in 1981 there was an incident in which some people became ill through inadequate teaching which subsequently created bad publicity for qigong. When qigong became popular in China many people set themselves up as qigong teachers when they had had very little real training in the exercises themselves. The Chinese government is now trying to control qigong teaching in China.

It is all too easy for Westerners to think that just because someone is Chinese they must be a good qigong teacher. Conversely, a Westerner may be well qualified to teach.

HOW DO I FIND A GOOD TEACHER?

As qigong grows in popularity there will be more and more qigong teachers appearing on the scene so it is important to find a good one.

The best way to know whether a tree is healthy is by the fruit it produces. The best way to tell whether teachers are competent is by the pupils they produce.

First we need to decide what kind of qigong we wish to practise. It is no use going to a teacher who is primarily teaching a martial art when what we really wanted was qigong for health maintenance. Many experienced teachers will teach qigong for a combination of uses which include a martial art and healing as well as spiritual development. A good way of finding out about a teacher is to talk to the pupils and find out about the benefits they reap from their practice. Another way is going to see the teacher to find out whether he or she seems trustworthy and therefore the teaching he or she is giving is sound. We can also find out about the teacher's track record and how long he or she has been teaching.

If all this seems good then go for it!

HOW MUCH DO I NEED TO PRACTISE?

For the maximum benefit it is best to do qigong every day. People who practise regularly notice the most beneficial effects. Most practise for at least half an hour every day, some practise for longer but it is still possible to feel beneficial results with less time devoted to doing the exercises as long as they are done regularly.

Regular practice is important for a number of reasons. One reason is that we need to have a routine. A regular routine means that we will continue to exercise through the difficult times as well as when it is easy. A second reason is that practising every day takes discipline and is also a way of developing strong mental power. A third reason is that regular practice also gives us something to build on. If we only do qigong intermittently we never build our energy and will find that we always go back to square one and never progress.

Here is an interesting comment from a mother of two children:

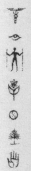

'For the last two years I have stopped doing qigong during the summer break due to a lack of personal space and my classes stopping. Each time I have found that at the end of the six weeks, in spite of going on holiday, I am a wreck – I feel exhausted and out of sorts. As soon as I start practising qigong regularly my vitality returns. Having made the mistake for two consecutive years I hope that I've learned my lesson.'

WHERE SHOULD I PRACTISE?

Although it is important to have a good teacher our actual day-to-day practice goes on at home. It is best to have a regular place to exercise. A quiet room or a special space in a room can make a regular routine easier to maintain.

Practising with a group is a very different experience from practising alone. The energy in the room is heightened by the presence of more than one person exercising their Qi. This in turn can improve the results of the practice. A good teacher will create an even stronger Qi 'field' in the group which can form the basis for many breakthroughs in qigong practice.

This chapter is a brief description of qigong. The proof of the pudding is in the eating and we have to practise the exercises in order to achieve the benefits described. Qigong is one way that we can take responsibility for our own health, especially when we have already obtained a better balance of Qi from having acupuncture, herbs or tui na massage. I know it's true. I use it myself.

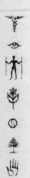

7

TUI NA,
CHINESE MASSAGE
TOUCHING YOUR ENERGY

A child falls over and bangs its knee. It cries in pain. Its mother instinctively rubs it better and this pacifies the distraught infant. The support from its mother's touch helps the child to quickly get over the trauma.

A colleague gets a headache – a tight, throbbing pain. She instinctively massages the area and easily finds pressure points to rub on her neck and temples. Kneading these points relieves the headache and she also finds it comforting.

A friend is in distress and tells her partner about the difficulties she has with her critical boss and her resulting lack of confidence. He feel compassion for her plight and reaches out to hold her hand as she talks. Holding her hand supports her and enables her to let her feelings out. She begins to feel renewed strength to cope with her difficulties.

To reach out and touch another person is a natural reaction when someone is in physical or mental distress. These are all examples of how touch can give a clear and direct message of caring, warmth, comfort or healing.

Chinese massage, known as *tui na*, is one of the oldest of the Chinese therapies. It was originally born from our instinct to make physical contact with someone in need of healing and support.

Although it is so old, it is still in its infancy in the Western world. In the UK there are only a small number of fully qualified practitioners. The good news is that the numbers are growing as more people are training to practise this method of treatment.

In this chapter we will look at all the questions that may be asked about this therapy including what happens during a treatment, the different ways tui na can be used and what it can treat. We will also examine how tui na is different from other forms of massage and in what way it uses the theory of Chinese medicine for diagnosis. We'll begin by discovering the nature of tui na.

WHAT IS TUI NA?

Tui na is Chinese therapeutic massage. It is currently used in many hospitals throughout China to cure a wide range of illnesses. Before the massage commences a patient has a full case history taken and is given a complete diagnosis.

The name 'tui na' actually means 'push grab'. This is a term that has been used since the Ming dynasty which began around the mid-14th century. Before that time all massage was called 'an mo' which means 'press rub'. The term 'an mo' now describes domestic or relaxing massage only.

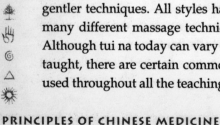

Therapeutic massage has a long and diverse history. Different styles developed in different regions of China. The northern areas of China are well known for their more vigorous style of massage and the southern regions for their fine and gentler techniques. All styles have their own unique uses and many different massage techniques have evolved from them. Although tui na today can vary slightly according to where it is taught, there are certain common massage techniques that are used throughout all the teaching centres in China and the West.

We will look at some of these techniques as this chapter progresses. Next, however, let us look at how tui na and other styles of massage compare.

WHAT IS THE DIFFERENCE BETWEEN TUI NA AND OTHER STYLES OF MASSAGE?

There are two main uses for massage. The first use is to relax a person and the second is to cure illness. Relaxing massage is most frequently practised in the West and a style called 'Swedish' massage is commonly taught. Swedish massage can be very useful when a person has tight muscles and tension, but it is not used to cure specific ailments. 'An mo' which was mentioned earlier is different from Swedish massage but is used in a similar way.

The second use of massage is to cure illness. A physiotherapist may apply forms of massage to ease joint and muscle problems, but no form of Western massage practised today is actually used to cure disease in the same way as tui na.

Another form of popular therapeutic massage used in the West is 'shiatsu' massage. Shiatsu massage which comes from Japan originated in China and was taken to Japan in the Tang dynasty which began in 618 AD. During this time in China, massage was carried out on the floor with the practitioner kneeling next to the patient. This part of the tradition continues in Japan to this day where shiatsu massage is still always carried out on the ground. In China these days most massage is practised on treatment couches which come up to waist height.

Some forms of shiatsu massage practised in Japan are still similar to tui na. There are many different traditions of shiatsu and most of those done in England and the US are similar to but are not the same as tui na. It has been 1,350 years since tui na was first taken to Japan so it would be surprising if they were still the same after all these years!

WHAT WILL HAPPEN WHEN I FIRST COME FOR TREATMENT?

When the patient first comes for treatment the practitioner will take a case history in order to clarify the diagnosis. She will be looking for the cause of the main problem as well as taking into consideration the overall health of the patient.

During the diagnosis the practitioner will ask many questions which will vary from 'How do you sleep?' to 'How is your appetite?' or 'How do you relax?' The practitioner will also take the twelve pulses on the wrist and look at the tongue (see chapter 2).

As one patient described, 'My practitioner asked me common sense questions really, she was getting to know all about me and my lifestyle.' Another said, 'The consultation made me think about my past illnesses and how they are connected with my health now.'

HOW IS THE THEORY OF CHINESE MEDICINE USED BY A PRACTITIONER OF TUI NA?

When taking a case history the masseur will be looking at three main areas.

First, the tui na practitioner will want to find out about the balance of the 'Vital Substances' in the body. The substances are the Qi, Blood, Body Fluids, Jing Essence and the Shen. These are mentioned in greater detail in chapter 1. The Qi and the Blood are the most important of these five Substances to the tui na practitioner. She will notice if the Qi and Blood are deficient or moving sluggishly in any parts of the body. Massage on the patient will naturally move the Qi and the Blood and will help to restore better health.

Secondly, the practitioner will also want to find out about the state of the internal organs and will later use massage to harmonize the Qi and Blood in these organs. For example massage techniques can be used to clear headaches which are created by imbalances in many organs including the Liver, back problems which have numerous causes including weakness of the Kidneys or even loose bowels which can be brought on by an imbalanced Spleen. The practitioner may then choose to treat points or energy pathways which are connected with these organs. These pathways are described in greater detail in chapter 4 on acupuncture.

Thirdly, the practitioner will be diagnosing any 'pathogens' in the body. Pathogens are Damp, Wind, Cold, Dryness or Heat. Their presence in the body can create many symptoms including colds and flus, some joint problems, stomach disorders or bowel complaints. Tui na can clear the pathogens when they cause obstructions. This will in turn free up the circulation of the Qi and Blood and can help the condition. Many joint problems are caused by these stuck pathogens being caught in the joints and tui na is especially beneficial in many of these disorders.

The tui na massage therapist will form a diagnosis based on her questioning and her observation of the patient. Having made the diagnosis she will then treat the patient.

WHAT ILLNESSES CAN TUI NA HELP?

Tui na is beneficial in relieving various joint problems. These may range from bad backs, painful shoulders, any joint problems of the arms and hands or legs and feet as well as helping neck problems or headaches. It can benefit both acute injuries or longer term, more chronic complaints.

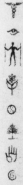

Tui na can also help a person to relax. Although it is not specifically used for relaxation, treatment does have the effect of relaxing a person both physically and mentally.

Although it is best known for its capacity to heal joint problems and create relaxation it can help any of the complaints listed in chapter 4 on acupuncture. These include digestive and bowel disorders, lung complaints, gynaecological problems, urinary diseases and acute infections.

BEVERLEY'S STOMACH IS CURED BY TUI NA

Beverley has every reason to be grateful to tui na for solving her stomach problems. She is 49 years old and works as a rep for a large drug company. She describes how she was before starting treatment.

> 'I had had stomach disorders for over 20 years and took many different medical drugs for the problem. None of them was really effective and the problem gradually became worse. By the time I went for tui na I had severe pain in my stomach that rose up to my breast bone and through to my back. The only thing that relieved the pain was being sick. When I was sick it came out in jets and I would also vomit blood as the blood vessels burst. It got to the stage when I was given a special phone number for an ambulance and if I rang they'd come and fetch me straight away. The doctors diagnosed me as having diverticulitis; then they thought it might be an ulcer or irritable bowel. When they wanted to cut out some of my gut I decided to try tui na.'

Beverley started treatment over a year ago and she is now completely cured of all her problems.

> 'I'm completely well now. I can do everything and I don't get any pain any more. I used to get such discomfort in my stomach that I even hated clothes being near the area and couldn't put my hands on my stomach at all. That's all gone now. After the first few treatments the sickness stopped and the stomach eased. Now I'm off all my drugs and I also feel

fantastic in my spirits. This treatment doesn't just treat one thing; it treats the whole person.'

Beverley's life has been transformed by having tui na treatment. Ironically she was voted 'rep of the year' by the drug company she works for last year, but is relieved that she no longer needs to take medical drugs in order to do her job well. For the future? She's decided to change her job and that she's going to train to use Chinese herbs.

WHAT WILL I EXPERIENCE DURING THE TREATMENT?

Having made a diagnosis the masseur will choose the treatment that is needed. Each individual's treatment will be designed differently according to the patient's energetic balance.

At treatment the patient lies down on the couch and the practitioner asks the patient how she has been since the previous treatment. She will also take the pulses and look at the tongue and check to see in which ways the patient has made progress since the last treatment. The practitioner will then begin the treatment. Often she will cover the area to be massaged with a towel. The patient does not usually need to remove clothing.

Here are some comments people have made to describe what it is like to have a treatment. A man aged 31 years says, 'It is really comfortable having the massage, if my back is a bit achy or in spasm it can hurt a little bit but that's unusual and it's usually very pleasant. The massage is quite vigorous and very effective.' Another 28-year-old patient states, 'I drift off. It feels wonderful. It's very fast and precise and I can feel the pain falling out of my body.' A 49-year-old woman has said, 'At first some areas hurt a lot and it was as if my practitioner could pick

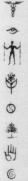

every sensitive place on my body, but as I've got better the pain is not as bad.'

WHAT ARE TUI NA MASSAGE TECHNIQUES LIKE?

Rolling, pushing, grasping, kneading, rubbing, nipping, vibrating, chopping, revolving, pinching and pressing are but a few names of the many tui na massage techniques that are commonly used.

Two massage techniques are used extensively and the tui na practitioner practises these for at least a year on a bag filled with rice or sand in order to competently master the technique.

The first of these techniques is called 'Gun Fa' (pronounced goon fa). This technique is a rolling technique. The back of the hand is rotated and rolled to and fro over the body using flexion and extension of the wrist. It is used for deep massage over large areas such as the lower back, shoulders or the thick muscles of the limbs. It can powerfully strengthen or relax areas of the body as well as clearing blockages and it is known to be remarkably penetrating in its effect.

The second technique is called 'Yi Zhi Chan' (pronounced ye je chan) which is translated as 'one finger oscillation'. To use this technique the practitioner presses on a chosen area using the tip of the thumb, at the same time she keeps the shoulder, elbow and wrist relaxed and moves the thumb inwards and outwards using flexion and extension. The result of using this technique is to create a potent and intense stimulus which can work directly on an acupuncture point when stimulation is needed. It is used for many of the medical problems that tui na can treat and is especially valuable on the abdomen for conditions such as abdominal, gastro intestinal and gynaecological diseases. It can be applied to very sensitive areas such as around the eyes and other sense organs as well.

By perfecting these two massage techniques tui na practitioners strengthen the muscles of their arms and hands and loosen their wrists. All of the other massage techniques spring from these two basic ones and once these movements have been mastered the other actions come naturally.

The massage techniques are used individually or combined together to create more sophisticated techniques. A practitioner will carefully choose the exact manoeuvre which is necessary for the patient and decide which areas to treat before beginning treatment.

WHAT AREAS OF THE BODY WILL THE PRACTITIONER TREAT?

Sometimes the tui na masseur will massage specific acupuncture points on the body, at other times she may treat along an energy pathway and on other occasions she may choose to massage a whole area of the body.

The practitioner may choose individual points because they are known to have a particular effect or because they lie on a pathway which is connected to an organ. For example, a patient with severe digestive problems was often treated using Stomach and Spleen channel points on the leg known as 'Stomach 36' and 'Spleen 6'. This was because of the nature of her illness and because the complaint had originated in her Stomach and Spleen organs. Sometimes, however, her practitioner would also use other points on different channels such as a Pericardium point on the arm called 'Pericardium 6' and 'Directing vessel 12' which lies over the Stomach area. She would choose these points as they were particularly beneficial for the specific complaint and would often use the 'one finger

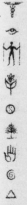

PRINCIPLES OF CHINESE MEDICINE

scillation' technique to massage the points.

A masseur may also decide to treat along a whole meridian pathway on the body rather than on an individual point. This may have a more generalized effect on the channel rather than the specific effect obtained from using individual points. For example a patient with a severe headache may have massage along the energy channels of the shoulders and neck as well as the head.

Sometimes the practitioner may massage a whole area on the body, such as the lower back area or the lower abdomen. One tui na patient aged 31 years is a futures trader in London. This work involves him standing on a pit in one spot for many hours at a time. He says, 'My back seizes up after a while. Treatment pummels the stress out of it and I feel much better and more relaxed afterwards. I want to continue, as it helps me mentally and physically.' Although tui na is not used merely for relaxation there are times when it is important to relax a whole area of the body for it to have its therapeutic effect.

WHAT SKIN PREPARATIONS WILL THE PRACTITIONER USE?

Western trained masseurs often use a massage oil directly on the skin. Chinese massage is different. Sometimes the practitioner will use a medium on the skin and sometimes not. One traditional way of carrying out a massage is to place a cotton cloth over the area being treated. This is a common practice and creates a flat area on which the massage is given.

If a medium is used on the skin it is chosen according to the diagnosis. For example, if a patient is too Damp, pure talcum powder can be used as it has a drying effect. If a condition needs to be warmed such as a cold achy back, then hot substances can be used on the area. These may be tiger balm, another balm called 'essential' balm or woodlock oil. Woodlock oil may be applied after a massage and it will deeply penetrate and warm an area at the finish of the treatment. One patient commented, 'She rubbed an oil into my lower back and I felt the warmth sinking into my bones.'

Dong Qin Gao (pronounced dong chin gow) is another oil which is frequently used. It has a Vaseline base and is made from wintergreen mixed with menthol. It is commonly used for lumbago or sciatica and is applied to large areas such as the back or the legs to move congested Qi and Blood.

Vinegar is often used on injuries and sprains and may be mixed into a paste with other substances such as jasmine and ginger. This clears swellings and relieves pain. Chinese herbs are also sometimes used on the skin to add to the effects of the massage.

WILL THE PRACTITIONER EVER MANIPULATE MY SPINE?

Yes, a fully trained tui na practitioner can manipulate the spine if it is essential for the patient's well being. The Chinese word for manipulation is 'Ban Fa'. The word 'Ban' means twisting and 'Fa' means technique.

A manipulation is only applied after a great deal of massage has been used and the whole area is thoroughly loosened up. Usually Ban Fa is used on the lower back although it can also be applied to the neck.

Often a displaced vertebra will automatically correct its position after a tui na treatment has been given so no manipulation will then be necessary. The muscles around the spine become relaxed and loosened after massage allowing the spine to naturally realign itself.

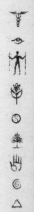

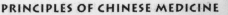

A CURE FOR TERRY'S BACK AFTER 20 YEARS

Terry decided to try tui na treatment after being impressed by how much it helped his wife. He'd had a fall over twenty years ago and had a back problem ever since.

'I'd had some osteopathy and it had temporarily relieved it for a few days but never on a long-term basis. The doctor had told me that I'd have to live with it. Most of the time I'd tried to ignore it as I thought I'd have it for the rest of my life. The problem was always there. It was a dull ache, on the right-hand side of my back and the pain also went to my hip and travelled down my leg. I'd wondered if I had anything wrong with my hip as well, but when my practitioner examined me she said that the main problem was in the lower back.

'The treatment itself was not uncomfortable, in fact I was nearly going to sleep sometimes while she was treating me. After the first treatment I felt slightly better, then after the second one I dramatically improved. The third treatment was just the finishing touches really and that was all I needed. I've had no problems since. Tui na was able to do for my back what nothing else could do – that is it has helped me on a permanent basis.'

Terry has been better for 6 months now and although he's had a few slight twinges his back has been fine. He still treats his back with respect and he does some exercises that his practitioner recommended because as he says, 'I think they help me to stay healthy.'

HOW LONG WILL A TUI NA TREATMENT TAKE?

A treatment will usually last from three quarters of an hour to one hour, but this depends on the nature of the problem that is being treated.

HOW OFTEN WILL I NEED TO COME FOR TREATMENT?

An acute condition will require more frequent treatments than a chronic one but fewer treatments will be needed overall. For example a patient with an acute sprained ankle may require treatments every other day but the problem can be cured in a short number of treatments.

A patient with a chronic problem such as long-term joint problems, digestive problems or period problems may initially need weekly treatments. These will be spread out to increasingly longer intervals such as fortnightly, monthly and two monthly as they get better.

A patient with a chronic complaint can expect to need more treatments before getting better than those with an acute complaint. The amount of treatment each person needs will vary from individual to individual and depend to some extent on their lifestyle as well as how long they have been ill and the treatments they have already had.

HOW WILL I FEEL IMMEDIATELY AFTER THE TREATMENT?

Here are some comments from the patients saying what they experience immediately after having tui na. 'I always came out feeling totally different, I had a feeling of lightness after treatment. After I came back I'd often go to sleep for a while it was so restful.' 'I felt centred and brought down to a very relaxing level, I also felt warm and almost maternal at times.' 'I'm so relaxed after the treatment I can hardly speak! My voice is a tone lower and I can hardly say anything for 2–3 hours. It relieves the pain and the stresses of the day.'

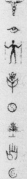

CAN TUI NA BE USED TO TREAT CHILDREN?

There is a long tradition in China of tui na being used to treat children. Children respond very quickly to massage treatment as their energy is usually strong and vibrant. Changes in health tend to be more immediate in the treatment of many conditions than when adults are treated. This is not to say that adults cannot also respond quickly to treatment. They do, however, tend to take longer to change than children as their energy has often become more depleted or blocked as life has taken its toll – some cynics may even add that sometimes it's having children that causes this depletion!

Children's tui na is slightly different from that used on adults and employs its own specific techniques. It is usually carried out on children under twelve years and is especially effective on infants under five. In China the tui na clinic is often the first port of call for children who are ill and treatment is used for a wide variety of complaints from asthma and infantile diarrhoea to paralysis due to polio.

The other bonus of using this treatment is that besides being effective, children usually enjoy the treatment. In some cases some treatment can be applied by caring relatives at home, once the masseur has directed them in what to do.

CAN I USE MASSAGE TECHNIQUES ON MYSELF?

Sometimes the tui na practitioner will instruct her patient on how to do a self-massage technique. The patient can then use it at home and it will support the treatment. This is especially useful when someone has an injury or more chronic musculo-skeletal disorders and when the area in need of treatment is

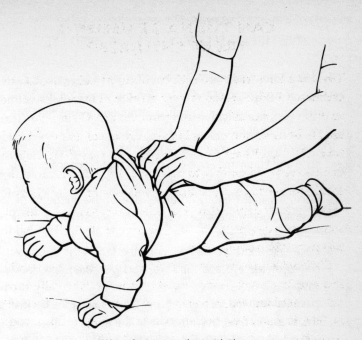

Tui na being used on a baby

easy to locate. She may also suggest exercises that can be practised daily in order to aid healing.

Although not specifically a tui na technique this exercise is taught to schoolchildren in China to relax their eyes when they do schoolwork. It is useful during or after any activity that may strain the eyes.

FIVE-MINUTE SELF-MASSAGE FOR TIRED EYES

1 Place thumbs level with the inner corner of the eyes at the side of the bridge of the nose. Rest the fingers on the forehead. Lightly massage in a circular motion towards the nose with the thumbs.

2 Place thumb and first finger on the side of the bridge of the nose and lightly massage in a circular motion concentrating on pulling downwards and releasing slightly.

3 Place first finger lightly on either side of the bridge of the nose and gently massage outwards following the line of the bone below the eye.

4 Place first finger in the hollow of the temple at the outer corner of the eye and massage clockwise then anti-clockwise.

5 Place the first and second finger in the hollow at the back of the neck which is below the base of the skull and about one and a half inches from the midline (the first prominent hollow). Press in on the point and massage clockwise then anti-clockwise.

To sum up, tui na is fast becoming a popular treatment and over time there will be many more practitioners available to give this therapy in order to restore health and to prevent disease. In the meantime we should keep our eyes and ears open as tui na receives more publicity and becomes as much a household name as acupuncture and Chinese herbs.

CHINESE DIETETICS
NOURISHING YOUR ENERGY

I first visited China in 1980 with a group of acupuncturists. As we travelled from city to city we attracted a lot of attention. Many Chinese people had never seen pale skin, blue eyes or blond hair before and they had no inhibitions about staring at us in great curiosity. One member of our group, Mary, drew more attention than all of us put together. She was overweight. It became clear that these people had never seen an obese person before.

Why is it that Chinese people rarely become overweight? Although there is less choice of food in China compared with the vast selection in the West, people eat simply and are well nourished. The answer is that Chinese people understand diet better than we do. By eating well, they naturally maintain their weight, as well as remain healthy.

There are so many dietary 'fads' coming and going here in the West that people often end up feeling confused about what constitutes a healthy diet. Many Western diets are devised especially to help people to lose weight without always considering whether they are healthy or not. These often cannot be sustained and people's weight can yo-yo. It makes more sense to eat a healthy diet and to lose weight slowly and naturally.

118   In contrast, basic dietary rules in China have not changed over thousands of years. Chinese dietary therapy does not follow a rigid regime although it will be adjusted according to a person's age, build, health and living conditions. This diet has stood the test of time and is based on sound principles.

There are five main dietary recommendations. If we can follow them we will be eating balanced and healthy meals and get the best possible nourishment from our food. They are:

1 The proportions of different types of food

2 The temperature

3 The taste

4 The quality of the food

5 How and when we eat our food

In this chapter we will look at each of these in turn. First let's look at how diet relates to Chinese medicine.

HOW DOES THE THEORY OF CHINESE MEDICINE APPLY TO DIET?

The stomach and spleen are the two main organs of digestion. We can care for and maintain these organs by eating well.

Chapter 31 of *The Classic of Difficulties* says: 'the *Stomach* is responsible for rotting and ripening food and drink.' This rotting and ripening process is the first step in the assimilation of what we eat. We need to send down digestible food to the Stomach at the correct temperature, at regular times and in the right quantities.

Cold food puts a strain on the Stomach. Too much cold food chills the body and the digestion is slowed down. The Stomach has to use extra energy to heat it up as *the process of digestion requires warmth*. A Chinese friend of mine was shocked by the American habit of drinking iced water even at breakfast. This strains the Stomach and Spleen to the extent that it can bring the digestive process to a standstill and cause many digestive problems as well as contributing to some people retaining water or becoming obese.

Insufficiently chewed or indigestible food will also put a burden on the Stomach which has to use up large quantities of energy to break the food down to a digestible liquid. The Chinese therefore put great emphasis on the *quality of the food* sent down to the Stomach to be digested.

After food has been rotted and ripened by the Stomach, the Spleen transforms and moves it. Each nutrient will ultimately become one of the Vital Substances such as Qi, Blood, Body Fluids, Jing Essence or Shen. This will in turn nourish us, both in our body and our mind-spirit. If the Spleen is functioning poorly or we eat badly this can cause tiredness, poor skin and hair quality, bowel problems, stomach aches, weak limbs and poor muscle tone. It can also influence us mentally and affect our concentration and memory. A weak Stomach and Spleen can lead us to start worrying and over-thinking.

Chinese medicine also recognizes the role of the Large and Small Intestine in the process of assimilating our food and drink, as does Western physiology. If they are weak this may result in digestive problems such as loose stools or constipation, rumbling bowels or bloating in the abdomen.

A weak Small or Large Intestine can also affect us mentally. If the Small Intestine function is weakened we may have difficulty 'separating pure from the impure' in our minds and have trouble making clear choices in our lives. If the Large Intestine is imbalanced we may be unable to excrete mental 'waste' and may hang on to old resentments and feelings. We may also har-

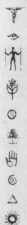

bour negative thoughts that are better discarded. A good diet is important for our health at all levels of our being.

WHAT ARE THE BEST PROPORTIONS OF GRAINS, PULSES, VEGETABLES, FRUIT AND MEAT IN THE DIET?

Chinese diets contain more grains, fruit and vegetables and less meat, sugar and fat than most Western diets. As a general measure of proportions, a diet should be made up of 40–60 per cent grains and pulses, 20–30 per cent fruit and vegetables and about 10–15 per cent meat, fat, seafood, and dairy produce. We will look at each of these in turn.

The Chinese consider rice to be the most nourishing *grain* to

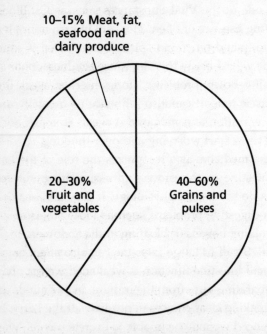

Pie chart of proportions of food

eat as it is neither too Hot nor too Cold. It also clears away Dampness. Dampness is formed when Body Fluids don't move through the body properly and it can generate symptoms such as retention of body fluids, heavy limbs, a bloated sensation in the abdomen as well as poor concentration, lethargy and a muzzy, heavy head. Other grains such as wheat, oats, barley and rye are also nutritious but tend to be more damp forming than rice. We can incorporate grains into our diets in the form of cooked grains, breads, noodles and porridges and include them in soups and stews.

Pulses include lentils, aduki beans, kidney beans, chickpeas, mung beans and tofu which is made from soya beans. Soya bean products and mung beans are both considered to be Cold foods and should be balanced with more Warming food.

Cooked *vegetables* are considered to be more easily assimilated by the body than raw ones. Because they are warm they also put less strain on the digestion than cold raw vegetables. Raw vegetables and fruit are also more eliminating whilst cooked ones are more building for the body. Anyone who is depleted in energy will benefit from eating cooked vegetables. It is best to eat organic and fresh vegetables and fruit, in order to gain the full benefit of the vitamins and minerals available from them. There will be a more detailed explanation of the difference between cooked and raw food later on in this chapter.

Meat and *dairy produce* are highly nutritious foods which are very rich in quality. Because of the high concentration of nourishment they contain the Chinese consider that they should only be eaten in small amounts and make up 10–15 per cent of the whole diet. Many Western diets are too heavily biased towards meat and dairy products with far too few cooked vegetables.

The result of eating too much meat is that the body can produce Damp and Heat. Some examples of heat symptoms are inflammations as well as aggression and irritability.

IS IT BETTER TO BE A VEGETARIAN OR A MEAT EATER?

It is becoming increasingly popular for people to become vegetarian. There are a number of reasons for this. One is that many people decide to stop eating meat on ethical grounds as they feel that it is incompatible with a meditative or religious lifestyle. A second reason is that people don't like to think of eating animals which have been badly treated or cruelly slaughtered and decide not to eat any meat as an expression of their feelings. A third reason for not eating meat is that some people say that it is healthier to be a vegetarian than to be a meat eater.

The Chinese would disagree with this last suggestion. A small amount of meat can be a vital constituent of many people's diet as the protein found in animal products helps to form the Blood in our bodies.

Blood deficiency can lead to insomnia, poor short-term memory, anxiety and jumpiness, cramps, pins and needles and brittle nails. Another symptom is a pale dull face. I read an article recently which said that many young girls had become vegetarian to make themselves look fashionably paler. I wonder if they would have been so keen on this diet if they had known the other effects it was having on their health.

In general a diet with a small amount of meat products is considered the healthiest. Some people have called this an *almost* vegetarian diet. About 2–3 ounces of meat 3–4 times per week is a good balance. If a person decides not to eat meat for religious or moral reasons then it is important that the rest of the diet is as well balanced as possible. The best vegetarian diets I know are ones which combine pulses and grains for protein, along with rice, lentils and vegetables.

The Chinese often cut their meat, fish or poultry into small strips and mix it with their rice or noodles. Vegetarianism in

China is rare. I was once told by a Chinese colleague that some people in China are now becoming vegetarians. He added that they often put gravy on their food in order to substitute for the meat!

PATRICIA'S DIETARY HEADACHE

Patricia looked tired and pale when she came for treatment. She was 18 years old and studying for her A levels.

> 'Sometimes I get headaches every day and then none at all. I last had some a fortnight ago and they went on continually. They're a constant dull ache usually across my forehead but occasionally all over my head. When I have them it's hard to concentrate on my studying. They often start in the middle of the day and I can go to bed with one and wake up with it again in the morning.'

She had very few other symptoms that she was aware of although her periods were rather scanty, her nails broke easily and she also occasionally felt light headed. The symptoms she related added up to a picture of 'Blood deficiency'. I wondered why this was happening. The answer was provided when she talked about her diet. On a normal day she described a diet of sandwiches, crisps and chocolate bars. A few cooked meals were thrown in and she ate very few vegetables.

Her diet had deteriorated when she became vegetarian 18 months ago. Before that she would join in with family meals. I let her know that improving her diet would make her feel better and combined with a little meat or fish it would 'strengthen her blood'. She was a little resistant to eating some meat or fish, although not morally opposed to it. She did however agree to try some.

She came to see me again a week later telling me, 'I'm not Blood deficient. I've had a blood test and my doctor says my red blood cell count is fine.' Like many people she had thought that the Chinese term 'Blood deficient' meant that she was anaemic. I explained that this was

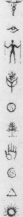

not the case and blood deficiency was determined by a pattern of signs and symptoms that a person has, not by a low blood count.

Armed with her new understanding she went away and decided that she would see what happened if she ate some meat as well as more vegetables for a while. Her headaches gradually improved. She reported feeling more energetic and that she could concentrate better on her studying. She got through her exams without having any headaches at all and decided to stay on her new diet and continue to eat a small amount of meat.

HOW IS THE TEMPERATURE OF FOOD IMPORTANT IN OUR DIETS?

As well as eating food in the correct proportions we can also take care over the temperature of the food we eat. This is the second important aspect of a healthy diet. The Chinese class all food as either 'Hot', 'Warm', 'Neutral', 'Cool', or 'Cold'. The term 'temperature' means the Warming or Cooling *effect* they have on the body rather than whether they are physically hot or cold.

Lamb, chocolate, eggs and butter are all heating or warming as are many foods which have a high fat content. Mangoes, bananas, grapes and bean sprouts are all Cooling or Cold as are many fruits or raw foods. The list in the box describes some of the most common foods and their temperatures.

By closely observing our bodies we can often tell if a food is more Heating or Cooling; for example, a friend of mine will sweat on his head if he eats garlic which is a warming food. A hot 'toddy' made from whisky, lemon and honey is a surefire way of heating us up so that we can sweat and eliminate a common cold from the body.

We can notice the effect of too much Cold food on our digestion which needs to be kept warm, for example, we may get a 'stomach upset' if we eat too much fruit, or stomach pains from drinking too much cold beer in the summer. A close colleague had loose bowels all through his student days; it was only when he later learned about Chinese medicine that he realized that it had been because of his diet. He had almost lived on yogurt during that time and said, 'I had thought that such vast quantities were good for me!' Like many of us he hadn't known that yogurt was an extremely Cold food.

In general it is better to eat foods which are neither too Hot nor too Cold in their nature. We can also endeavour to balance the Hot and Cold foods we eat. Eating too much Hot food will give us health problems concerned with Heat which may be headaches, bloodshot eyes, night sweats and generally feeling physically Hot and 'hotter' tempered. Eating too much Cold or Cooling food can often affect the digestion and cool down the stomach giving us bloating, stomach pains, diarrhoea, cold limbs and even period pains in women if the lower abdomen gets too Cold.

If we eat extremely Hot food we can balance it with more Cooling food and vice versa. We can also balance our food according to the climate, a warming soup or stew will nourish us on a cold winter's day especially if it has a small amount of ginger added, whilst fruit can be far more appetizing in extremely hot weather.

SHOULD WE EAT COOKED OR RAW FOOD?

It has been suggested that eating raw food is one of the best ways to get all of the nutrients we need from our diet. The Chinese would not agree. They maintain that we should lightly cook most of our food. Raw food is Cold and is also less digestible. Digesting cold raw food takes more heat and energy from the stomach than warm cooked food. Raw food if

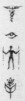

PRINCIPLES OF CHINESE MEDICINE

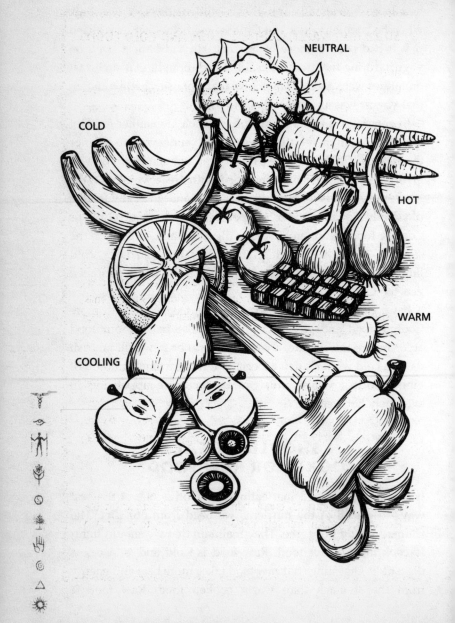

NEUTRAL

COLD

HOT

WARM

COOLING

PRINCIPLES OF CHINESE MEDICINE

SOME HOT, WARM, NEUTRAL, COOL AND COLD FOODS

HOT
Black pepper, butter, chicken fat, chocolate, coffee, crispy rice, curry, hot chillis, lamb, mango, onions, peanut butter, sesame seeds, smoked fish, trout, whisky.

WARM
Beef, brown sugar, cheese, chestnuts, chicken, egg yolks, dates, garlic, ginger, green pepper, ham, leeks, oats, peach, pomegranate, potato, turkey, turnip, walnuts, vinegar, wine.

NEUTRAL
Aduki beans, apricots, beetroot, black tea, bread, broad beans, brown rice, cabbage, carrots, cauliflower, cherries, chickpeas, egg white, grapes, honey, hot water, kidney beans, milk, oysters, peanuts, peas, plum, pork, raisins, salmon, sugar, sweet potatoes.

COOL
Almonds, apples, asparagus, barley, broccoli, cauliflower, celery, chicory, corn, fish, mushrooms, mango, mung beans, oranges, pears, pineapple, radishes, rhubarb, salt, seaweed, spinach, strawberries, tangerines, turnip, watermelon, wheat, wild rice.

COLD
Banana, beansprouts, cucumber, duck, grapefruit, green tea, lettuce, ice cream, mussels, peppermint, sorbet, tofu, tomato, water melon, yogurt.

analyzed scientifically may be found to be higher in certain nutrients such as vitamin C than food which has been cooked but this does not mean that this extra nourishment is assimilated better by the body during the process of digestion.

A patient told me that he was worried about his daughter who was going through a 'nervous breakdown' and I agreed to see her without delay. The daughter who was 25 years old told me, 'I started eating a raw food diet 6 months ago. At the time I felt better and had much more energy.' She had started the diet in June when it was warm. By December she didn't feel well. It was a very cold winter and she was still eating mainly uncooked food. When I saw her in February she was hardly coping with her life at all: 'I have no energy and I keep bursting into tears at the slightest difficulty.' I advised her to change her diet immediately. She started eating more balanced quantities of food as well as cooking it and over some months gradually regained her health and equilibrium.

Another 30 year old female patient complained, 'I feel the cold very badly'. She was surprised when I suggested that she should stop eating salads and change to cooking her vegetables. Her reaction was a mixture of surprise and relief. 'I've been trying to eat salads every day as I was told they were good for me but I've never really enjoyed them.' My suggestion made her realize that she instinctively preferred to eat Warmer food. Many people are similar to her and if they listen to their bodies they will naturally change to a more balanced diet.

HOW ARE THE FLAVOURS OF FOOD IMPORTANT FOR MAINTAINING OUR HEALTH?

The flavour of our food is the third major aspect to consider in our diet. There are five main flavours of food which are *Bitter*,

Sweet, *Sour*, *Pungent* and *Salty*. Many foods have two tastes, for example, vinegar is both Bitter and Sour, barley is both Salty and Sweet and turnip is a combination of Pungent and Bitter.

Sweet is the flavour that affects the Stomach and Spleen. A certain amount of a mild Sweet taste will benefit our digestion and tonify our Qi energy. The Chinese consider many foods such as rice, chicken, cabbage and carrots to have a sweet taste and to be nourishing. This mild and Sweet taste is very different from the taste of sweet associated with chocolate and candy.

People frequently crave chocolates and sweets because their stomach and spleen have been weakened. A small amount of mildly Sweet-tasting food will strengthen the Stomach and Spleen, whilst extremely Sweet foods will further weaken them. This creates a vicious circle of craving more and more sweet foods whilst the Stomach and Spleen become increasingly feeble. We already know that the Stomach and Spleen are in charge of transforming all of our food and drink in order to nourish us. A weak Stomach and Spleen cannot carry this out and this can result in malnutrition and very deficient Qi energy.

Frequently people are advised to avoid Salt in their diet. Salt is the taste connected with the Kidneys, which is understandable as it regulates the amount of moisture in the body and one function of the Kidneys is to balance the body's Fluids. An excessive amount of salt in the diet is not appropriate as this will deplete the functioning of the Kidneys especially if a person retains fluids. A small amount of salt on the other hand can be beneficial if a person is too Dry as it will encourage moisture in the body.

In general it is best to have a balance of all the flavours in the diet without eating any of them in excessive amounts. If we crave a certain taste in food this may be an indication that the associated organ is out of balance. A small amount of the food may enhance the functioning of that organ. Large quantities may make the imbalance more extreme.

FLAVOURS OF FOOD AND THEIR ASSOCIATED ORGANS

BITTER (HEART AND SMALL INTESTINE)
Alfalfa, asparagus, beer, broccoli, chicory, celery, coffee, grapefruit rind,lettuce, radish, raspberry leaf, tea, turnips, vinegar, watercress.

SWEET (STOMACH AND SPLEEN)
Aduki beans, apples, apricots, barley, beef, beetroot, cabbage, carrots, celery, cheese, cherries, chicken, chickpeas, coffee, courgettes, corn, cucumber, dates, grapes, grapefruit, honey, kidney beans, lamb, lettuce, malt, mandarins, mung beans, mushrooms, oranges, milk, oats, peaches, peanuts, pears, pineapples, plums, pork, potatoes, radishes, raspberries, rice, spinach, strawberries, sugar, tomatoes, walnuts, wheat, wine.

PUNGENT (LUNG AND LARGE INTESTINE)
Black pepper, cayenne pepper, chilli, cloves, cumin, garlic, green peppers, horseradish, leeks, marjoram, mint, mustard, nutmeg, peppermint, radishes, rosemary, soya oil, turnips, watercress, wheatgerm, wine.

SALTY (KIDNEY AND BLADDER)
Barley, crab, duck, garlic, ham, kelp, lobster, millet, mussels, oysters, pork, salt, sardines, seaweed.

SOUR (LIVER AND GALL BLADDER)
Aduki beans, apples, apricots, blackberries, blackcurrants, cheese, crabapples, gooseberries, grapes, grapefruit, green leafy vegetables, lemons, lychees, mandarin oranges, mangoes, olives, peaches, pears, pineapples, plums, pomegranates, raspberries, sour plums, strawberries, tomatoes, trout, tangerines, vinegar.

HOW CAN WE MAKE SURE THAT THE FOOD WE EAT IS OF GOOD QUALITY?

We know that we can eat a healthy diet simply and easily by balancing the proportions of grains and beans, vegetables and fruit and meat, and that we can adjust the temperature and tastes of our food according to our needs. We will now consider the fourth of the five main aspects of our diet, which is to eat good quality food. Here are some simple guidelines about the quality of the food we eat.

We can endeavour to eat pure fresh food whenever possible, to take food which is in season and grows in our own area and to eat a wide variety of foods. We shall discuss each of these in turn.

The 20th century has brought about the bulk production of food. Crops are sprayed with chemicals, animals are injected with drugs and both are produced on a mass scale instead of cared for on small farms. We have easy access to a huge variety of foods which were unobtainable to previous generations. They ate the simple foods which grew around them. It is impossible and unnecessary to reverse this process of change but the broad rules that we can follow are the same as in the past.

In general eat vegetables and meat which are organic or home grown, fresh and in season. Many supermarkets now sell organic food and there are increasing numbers of local organic farms. It is horrifying to realize that an apple has probably been sprayed over 26 times in its short life or that with much of the meat we eat we are also eating hormones, antibiotics and other chemical additives!

We can also avoid food that is over processed. You may be surprised to know that frozen peas have added sugar only to 'enhance' the taste and oranges are often injected with colour so that they 'look' nice.

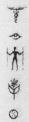

We can avoid an excess of any one food in the diet. It is natural to eat some foods such as grains and vegetables regularly, especially a particular vegetable which is in season. It is less useful to eat one food excessively even if it is good for us in small quantities. For example, an occasional orange might be very healthy but an excess of oranges in the diet or in the form of juices can encourage the formation of phlegm in the chest. A small amount of coffee can be a special 'treat'. Large amounts taken throughout the day can cause us to become overstimulated. In this state we override our body's messages telling us to stop when we need to rest. Short term we get much work done. Long term we may become exhausted and drain our reserves of energy. We then need even more coffee to keep us going. The end result of this lifestyle can be severe health problems.

If we eat these 'strong' foods in small amounts and more Neutral foods in larger amounts we will feel healthier mentally as well as physically. Many hyperactive children calm down if they have sugar and food additives cut out of their diets. Balancing our diets as adults can also have far reaching effects and allow us to become more settled and peaceful inside. How we feel inside is also affected by the *way* we eat our meals.

HOW IS IT BEST TO EAT OUR FOOD?

The last of the five aspects of good dietary practice is how and when to eat our food.

Many people eat their lunches as they walk along the streets while shopping or going about their business. It is even common for snack bars to have tables where people stand to eat – this is presumably better for business as it gives a quicker turnover than if seating is provided! 'Eating on the run' is a bad Western habit that leads us to eat overstimulating foods because we don't take the time to sit and let a simple diet nourish us properly. If we follow these rules we will get more nourishment from our food.

First, we really need to *relax* while we eat and *give our digestion time*. It is best to eat in pleasant relaxing surroundings. This is not always possible for those who have small children or busy lives but we can avoid overstimulating circumstances such as eating while watching the television or reading. It is best to give our food our full attention, to take the time to sit down and eat our meal and to allow time after eating for digestion to take place. The Chinese will often take 2 hours for their lunch, eat at a leisurely pace and even take a short nap after eating.

Secondly, we need to *chew our food* thoroughly. There is a saying that we should 'drink our food and chew our drinks'. If we chew our food until it becomes a fluid it will aid the first stage of digestion which is in the mouth. Here the saliva starts to break down the food which then gets passed on to the stomach in a predigested state. Allowing ourselves time to eat will remind us to chew our food thoroughly and enhance our digestion.

Thirdly, it is best *not to drink too much* while we are taking our meals. If we chew our drink we will take it in small amounts. Drinking too much at mealtimes swamps the digestion and washes our food down rather than allowing it to be thoroughly 'rotted and ripened'. A small warm drink can be taken a little before the meal and our main fluids between meals when we are not digesting our food.

Fourthly, it is a good idea to *eat until we are 75 per cent full*. This will allow our Stomach and Spleen to digest their contents thoroughly. If we overeat and then feel full and bloated we are straining these organs and food will sit in the Stomach for too long. This will in turn make us feel tired after the meal as we are using extra energy for digestion.

To sum up, it is best for us to eat our food without distractions and to give ourselves time to digest it properly. If we

134 chew our food thoroughly this will help the process of digestion. Sipping only a small amount of warm liquid before eating and nothing during meal times will allow the food to be digested properly rather than washed down. Finally we only need to eat until we are 75 per cent full so that the Stomach and Spleen don't have too much to assimilate.

WHEN IS IT BEST TO EAT?

It is best to eat at regular times. The Stomach likes regularity. Sometimes we have to miss a meal or eat at an unusual time if an unexpected situation arises, but this is preferably the exception rather than the rule.

There is a saying that we should 'eat breakfast like a king, lunch like a prince and supper like a pauper'. If we eat well at the beginning of the day it will set us up with enough energy to last through the morning. If we don't eat any breakfast we can become exhausted well before lunchtime and our blood sugar will drop. People often crave something sweet like cakes or chocolate bars to get a quick energy boost when they feel this drop. These will then overstimulate the Stomach if they are eaten regularly.

If we eat heavy meals very late at night our digestive system will be actively digesting food when we should be sleeping. This may result in insomnia or vivid dreams and we then don't feel rested when we wake in the morning. On the whole it is best that we eat our last meal of the day in the early evening so that our food is digested before we go to bed.

WHAT FOODS CAN I AVOID FOR SPECIFIC HEALTH PROBLEMS?

Following a healthy diet in the way that is described in this chapter, that is by eating the correct proportions of food and

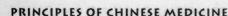

balancing the temperatures and tastes, will usually be enough to keep us in reasonable health.

For severe health problems it may be advisable to see a practitioner of one of the branches of Chinese medicine described in the other chapters of this book. Treatment with herbs, acupuncture, massage or qigong can then be supplemented with a healthy diet for the maximum effect from the treatment.

There are some foods that we can avoid so that we can gently shift the balance of our health in a positive direction.

If we are *too Hot* we can avoid foods that will heat us up. These include red meats, curries, greasy foods, alcohol and coffee. Other foods are listed in the 'Hot' and 'Warm' section of the box giving the temperatures of food. We will know if we are too Hot by our symptoms. These may include feeling hot all over or on our hands, feet and chest, also symptoms of bleeding such as nose bleeds or excessive uterine bleeding, hot flushes, restlessness, dry red eyes, night sweats or a red face. A person may also be prone to getting angry or irritable.

Cooling foods can be avoided if we are *too Cold*. These include any food taken straight from the refrigerator as well as raw vegetables and fruit, mung beans and soya produce. Other 'Cold' or 'Cooling' foods are mentioned in the box on food temperatures. If we are too Cold we may become more listless and tired, feel the cold very easily and even get numb extremities in cold weather. We may also get aches and pains such as joint, stomach, abdominal or period pains, which feel better with the application of heat.

If we have too much *Dampness* or *Phlegm* we may get symptoms such as oedema, swelling and bloating, poor concentration, heavy limbs or a muzzy head. Foods which should be avoided are dairy products which create mucus in the system, greasy food such as french fries or fatty meats, peanuts, concentrated fruit juices especially orange juice and tomato juice, and also sugary foods.

ARE THERE ANY FOODS THAT I CAN INCLUDE IN MY DIET FOR SPECIFIC HEALTH PROBLEMS?

If we are *too Dry* we may have symptoms such as dry skin, or any extreme dryness in other body parts such as the eyes, lips or throat. To remedy this imbalance we can include 'wetter' food in our diets such as sauces, stews and porridge. If on the other hand we are *too wet* or have *Damp* symptoms we can eat drier food and cook our food by grilling or baking.

It is also possible to include small amounts of heating foods in our diet if we are *too Cold*, such as adding a little ginger to our morning porridge or garlic to our soups and stews. We can add Cooling foods if we are *too Hot*, the Chinese consider mung bean soup a Cooling meal on a hot summer's day and soya produce is also very Cooling. Very Hot or Cold foods should only be taken in small quantities – it is better to stick with Warm or Cool foods. We also need to include lots of neutral foods to keep our diets balanced.

If we are *deficient in Blood* with symptoms such as poor memory, excessive anxiety, a pale dull face, scanty periods or pins and needles or cramps from poor circulation, then we need to eat more 'Blood forming' foods. The most common of these are animal products such as meat, poultry and fish. Leafy green vegetables and beans are also helpful as well as dates, apricots and figs.

CHRISTINE STOPS DAIRY PRODUCE

Christine is 43 years old and an acupuncturist. Looking at her now it is hard to believe that she was permanently ill until her mid-twenties. A change in her diet restored her health and created an interest in alternative medicine.

'I was a district nurse and I was permanently exhausted and depressed, in fact I had been like that for as long as I could remember. I also had very loose bowels and discomfort in my abdomen and every time I ate I got palpitations. I decided to go to my doctor who suggested that I saw a cardiologist. Frightened by this I looked around for something else. Fortunately a colleague suggested that I tried cutting out dairy produce.

'Within three weeks everything had changed completely, my heart had stopped pounding, my bowels improved and best of all my energy was wonderful. I was enjoying activities like swimming that I had never done before. Everything about my work and life shifted in perspective. I'd been so gloomy and flat and now I was enjoying my life like never before and it has continued to this day'.

In time Chris decided to train to become an acupuncturist. She now has a large thriving practice.

'From the perspective of Chinese medicine my symptoms were caused by a weak Stomach and Spleen which couldn't digest the milk leading to a milk "allergy". With hindsight I think I would have gone on to get a serious bowel disease if I hadn't changed my diet at that time'.

HOW SHOULD I GO ABOUT CHANGING MY DIET?

To recap, the five main aspects of eating healthily are eating the correct proportions of food, balancing hot and cold food and eating lots of neutral foods, including many tastes in our diet, eating good quality food and remembering the best times and conditions in which to eat.

The best method of making lasting changes is to make them slowly. A rapid change will often just as rapidly reverse itself and old habits definitely do die hard. We can look at our diets thoroughly and decide which healthy foods can easily be included. This will often involve taking more cooked vegetables

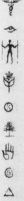

and grains. Once we have included good new habits in our diets, the bad old ones will often naturally drop away. If they don't we can decide to reduce unhealthy foods slowly until we have cut them out.

Sometimes it is best to go to a practitioner of Chinese medicine to get advice about changing our diet. The practitioner will then give support while the changes are being made.

WILL CHANGING MY DIET BE ENOUGH TO RESTORE MY HEALTH?

This may depend on a number of factors, the main one being whether a bad diet is the root cause of our ill health. If it is, then a change of our diet will improve our health substantially. Often, dietary changes will *maintain* good health in a patient who has been helped by acupuncture, herbs or massage treatment. It will also help the process of change to better health if used alongside other treatments.

We are in charge of what we eat. By eating well we can take responsibility for our own well-being. 'When is the right time to change my diet?' you might ask. The answer is, start *right now*.

WHICH ONE SHALL I CHOOSE?

THE RIGHT TREATMENT FOR ME

A friend read the transcript of this book. She came to me saying, 'Wow! I'm so excited by Chinese medicine. I'd like to have some treatment. Each treatment I read about is the one I'd like to try. So how do I decide which one to choose?'

This last chapter is dedicated to letting you and her know how to choose a practitioner for yourselves.

HOW DO I DECIDE WHETHER I NEED TREATMENT?

In this age of pollution, industrialization and fast living everyone can benefit from some form of treatment if they wish to have it. None of us can completely escape the consequences of life in the late-20th century. Even living close to nature in the heart of the countryside we can't avoid pollution.

Wind, Cold, Damp, Dryness and Heat – these external causes of disease can still affect us too. Internal causes of disease such as sadness, grief, anger or fear could have caused us distress in recent years or during our childhood and still be negatively influencing our health. We may decide that now is the time to deal with them.

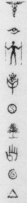

Having said this, some people need treatment more than others and people who generally feel well may prefer to look after their health by caring for their diet and exercising regularly.

People go for treatment for different reasons. Some have specific symptoms for which they would like help, other people don't have a 'named condition' but still benefit from treatment. Others have treatment in order to stay well or even prevent disease. The nature of Chinese diagnosis is to look for the cause of a problem and not merely to deal with named complaints so treatment can help in any of these varying circumstances.

Here are some different reasons why people decided to try Chinese medicine: 'I knew that if I didn't act now I would be put on strong medicines and I decided to try and avoid them.' 'I went to my doctor complaining that I felt tired and unwell. He said there was nothing wrong with me. I felt as if I was making it up. I was so relieved when my acupuncturist said that something could be done for me.' 'When I decided to try herbs it was really a last resort. I don't know what I would have done if they hadn't worked.' 'I didn't have much wrong with me but I was clear that my health was important and I wanted to remain well.'

SO WHICH TREATMENT SHALL I CHOOSE?

We may decide to have a particular treatment for one of many reasons: we may have a preference for that treatment; the treatment may be available to us in our area; we may think a particular treatment can help us best; or a particular practitioner may have been recommended. We'll talk about each of these in turn.

First, we may have a *preference for a particular type of treatment*. The best treatments to choose are the ones to which we are attracted. Having read this book we may feel excited by the idea of being treated by acupuncture, curious about tui na, intrigued by qigong or fascinated by Chinese herbs. If we do feel a strong pull towards a particular treatment that's the one to choose – but that is assuming it is available ...

Secondly, we also need to consider *what is available to us*. It is no use choosing to have tui na if we can't find a practitioner nearby. At present there are many more people qualified in acupuncture than in any of the other forms of Chinese medicine. This is partly because acupuncture was the first Chinese treatment for which training was available in the West and also because it is a very effective treatment. Most, although by no means all, herbalists are also qualified acupuncturists. There are very few tui na practitioners in the UK at present although the numbers are increasing. Although qigong practitioners are often centred in the cities rather than in small towns their numbers are growing too. Dietary advice can usually be obtained from any practitioners of Chinese medicine.

Thirdly, one reason for having a particular treatment is that we *think it can help us the best*. Different treatments certainly have a reputation for treating specific conditions. We may already know that acupuncture is well known for treating joint problems, arthritis and headaches and other kinds of pain. Any practitioner of acupuncture will tell you, however, that acupuncture is a wonderful treatment for countless other complaints including emotional and mental problems, digestive disorders, gynaecological complaints, fatigue and general weakness, as well as being used as a preventative treatment.

The same goes for treatment using herbs which have gained a reputation for treating skin disorders, gynaecological complaints and improving general deficiency disorders with great success. A herbalist might be proud to tell you of all of the other problems she has treated such as joint problems, allergies, bowel complaints, chest conditions and many other disorders.

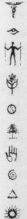

The list of conditions that each branch of Chinese medicine can treat is endless and the distinction between which treatment is best for which disorder is blurred. Once more it is not so much a question of which condition a treatment can help, as whether this treatment can help this particular patient?

A fourth reason why we might choose a particular treatment is because *a practitioner has been recommended to us*. There is nothing like hearing that a particular practitioner has helped someone else to convince us of the efficacy of that treatment and the practitioner. This is always a good way of deciding on where to have treatment.

In general it is best to use acupuncture, herbs, tui na or qigong healing when we are already ill. The help of a caring practitioner can be very important when we are going through difficult times and to coax us back to health.

Qigong exercises and a good diet will support us while we are having treatment, as well as once we have regained our health. If we decide on qigong or dietary therapy it is best to go to classes or to get good advice to start us off.

WHAT IS THE BEST WAY TO FIND A GOOD PRACTITIONER?

The best way to find a good practitioner is by word of mouth. We can ask around amongst our friends, colleagues and acquaintances to find out who has a good reputation in our area. Some clinics of complementary medicine are well known and can be recommended for having high quality practitioners who give first-rate treatment. Before going to any practitioner make sure they are properly qualified.

If there is nobody around to recommend a practitioner, the next best way is to ring the societies mentioned at the back of this book to find a practitioner nearby.

Another way of finding a practitioner is to look in the local phone directory but *only* if the practitioner is listed as a member of a professional body. If they are not, beware, as they may not be properly qualified. Adverts in bold type do not show who is well qualified. Practitioners are now allowed to advertise in newspapers, but this does not guarantee that all adverts are from well-qualified practitioners.

HOW CAN I TELL IF MY PRACTITIONER IS WELL QUALIFIED?

Make sure that your practitioner is registered with a recognized professional body. Members are bound by the Code of Ethics and Code of Practice of that society which will maintain high standards of discipline and health and safety to protect the general public. Practitioners of acupuncture, herbs or tui na who are members of a society have been well trained over a three or four year period.

A practitioner who is properly qualified will diagnose the patient thoroughly at the first appointment. She will ask many questions about the patient's health and other important areas of her life. She will also feel the twelve pulses at the wrist and look at the patient's tongue. If necessary she will also examine her spine or joints and feel for any temperature variations on her body.

Qigong is different. To tell if a qigong teacher is well qualified a person can ask him or her who they trained with and their 'lineage' of teachers. A lineage is the traditional line of teachers that have passed on their knowledge from teacher to student. It is also advisable to ask the other students in the group how they have benefited from the practice.

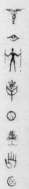

HOW CAN I TELL THAT THIS PRACTITIONER IS RIGHT FOR ME?

It is crucial that we trust in our practitioner's ability to help us. We don't have to believe in any of the treatments for them to work – in fact they can all be used successfully on animals or children – but treatment tends to progress faster if the patient feels safe in the care of her practitioner.

Some practitioners will talk to their patients more than others and patients themselves each prefer different amounts of conversation. No matter whether we discuss our condition and other health needs or not, another essential ingredient of successful treatment is good rapport. The patient might ask herself, 'Do I like this practitioner and feel she likes me?' One old traditional doctor described it as essential for a practitioner a have a 'good heart'.

Some comments patients have made about their practitioner are: 'She made me feel comfortable when I talked to her and I knew without doubt that she could help me.' 'I felt an immediate sense of "I can trust this person" and I felt the same way throughout treatment.' 'I felt great empathy from him, I think he understood.' 'I've been to three practitioners. They've all been very different and have helped me in different ways.'

SHOULD I CONSULT MY DOCTOR BEFORE GOING TO A PRACTITIONER?

Although it is unnecessary for the patient to tell the doctor that she is receiving treatment there is no harm in letting him or her know. If, however, a patient is taking medication or is under the constant care of her doctor then it is advisable to inform the doctor of her intentions.

Most doctors now welcome the idea of their patients trying

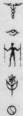

one of these complementary treatments. Twenty years ago when I first started practising acupuncture many doctors actively told their patients not to have treatment and as a result patients would often lie to their doctors or at least not mention their 'alternative' treatment. The climate has changed radically in a comparatively short space of time.

WHAT IF I AM ALREADY TAKING PRESCRIBED DRUGS FOR MY CONDITION?

A practitioner of Chinese medicine is trained to understand the effects of medication and will only ask a patient to reduce her drugs when she is ready and if it is appropriate. Drugs are usually reduced slowly as the patient's health improves. If the patient is on strong medication this is preferably carried out with the full co-operation of her doctor. Treatment will continue for as long as the patient needs it. In some cases coming off drugs can take a long time and the support of the practitioner can be helpful. Patients may never come off some 'replacement' drugs such as insulin for diabetes or vitamin B_{12} for pernicious anaemia but can still benefit from treatment with Chinese medicine.

HOW CAN I KEEP MYSELF HEALTHY?

Once a patient has regained her health many practitioners will suggest that she continue to have treatment at the change of season in order to keep her energy strong. A healthy lifestyle is also advisable. A good diet, a positive attitude in all situations and regular exercise will also support her health.

Exercising can become a valuable routine in a person's life. When I visited China and Hong Kong I was surprised by the number of Chinese men and women who regularly exercised

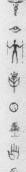

146 every morning in order to keep well. Many people practised qigong or other health exercises every day in the parks or in their homes before starting work. This was followed by a healthy breakfast to set them up for the day's work.

Eating healthily means being careful about our diet without being rigid. We can strive to carry out the guidelines suggested in chapter 8 on diet.

Finally, a *positive attitude* will go a long way in keeping us healthy. As Confucius said,

> If I were to sum up my whole philosophy in one sentence I should say: allow no negativity into your thoughts.

When life presents us with adversities, it is not always easy to find the 'positive lessons' that come from those situations, especially when they are painful. There are *always* things we can learn, however, and finding them rather than hanging on to bitterness or regrets can change a destructive attitude which leads to poor health into one from which we can grow and change and consequently become healthier.

A FINAL THOUGHT

By the time you have read this book you will have a good overview of Chinese medicine and its possible effects in treatment. If we respect and care for ourselves we are capable of leading long, happy, high-quality lives. The Chinese have a saying which translates as, 'good health is the root of happiness'. They also say, 'Even a journey of one thousand miles begins with a single step'. We can decide to take that step now – so that we can be empowered to take our good health into our own hands. I hope you enjoy your journey.

USEFUL ADDRESSES

I f you wish to find out more about any of these treatments you can ring the societies listed below.

UK

ACUPUNCTURE
British Acupuncture Council, Park House, 206 Latimer Road, London W10 2RE. Telephone 0181 964 0222

HERBS
Register of Chinese Herbal Medicine, PO Box 400, Wembley, Middlesex HA9 9NZ. Telephone 0181 904 1357

TUI NA MASSAGE
Register of Chinese Massage Therapy, PO Box 8739, London N28 DG.

QIGONG
Shen Hongxun Buqi Institute, c/o Sofie-Ann Bracke, 28 Brookfield Mansions, 5 Highgate West Hill, London N6 6AT. Telephone 0181 347 9862.

Tse Qigong Centre, PO Box 116, South PO, Manchester M20 3YN. Telephone 0161 434 5289.

Zhi Xing Wang and Wu Zhendi, Flat 3, 15 Dawson Place, London W2. Telephone 0171 229 7187.

If you wish to find out more information from the author you can contact her at the College of Integrated Chinese Medicine, 19 Castle Street, Reading, Berkshire RG1 7SB. Telephone 01734 508880.

AUSTRALIA

ACUPUNCTURE

Acupuncture Association of Victoria, 126 Union Road, Surrey Hills, Victoria 3127, Australia. Telephone 61 395 322 480.

Australia Acupuncture Ethics and Standards Organisation, PO Box 84, Merrylands, New South Wales 2160, Australia. Telephone 1800 025 334.

Australian Traditional Medicine Society, 120 Blaxland Road, Ryde, New South Wales, 2112 Australia. Telephone 809 6800.

HERBS

The National Herbalists Association of Australia, PO Box 61, Broadway NSW 2007, Australia. Telephone and fax 02 211 6452.

QIGONG

Qigong Association of Australia, 458 White Horse Road, Surrey Hills, Victoria 3127. Telephone 03 836 6961.

CANADA

ACUPUNCTURE

The Canadian Acupuncture Foundation, Suite 302, 7321 Victoria Park Avenue, Markham, Ontario L3R 278 Canada.

QIGONG

Master Shou-Yu Liang, Shou-Yu Liang Wushu Institute, 7951 No 4 Road, Richmond, BC, Canada V6Y 2T4. Telephone 604 228 3604/604 273 9648.

NEW ZEALAND

ACUPUNCTURE
New Zealand Register of Acupuncture, PO Box 9950, Wellington 1, New Zealand. Telephone 04 8016400.

QIGONG
David Hood, 341 Centaurus Road, Saint Martins, Christchurch 2, New Zealand. Telephone and fax 03 337 2838.

USA

ACUPUNCTURE
Council of Colleges of Acupuncture and Oriental Medicine, 1424 16th Street NW, Suite 501, Washington DC 20036. Telephone 202 265 3370.

National Acupuncture and Oriental Medicine Alliance, 1833 North 105th Street, Seattle, Washington DC 98133. Telephone 206 524 3511.

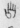

National Commission for the Certification of Acupuncturists, 1424 16th Street NW, Suite 501, Washington DC 20036. Tel 202 332 5794.

American Herb Association, PO Box 1673, Nevada City, California 95959. Telephone 916 265 9552.

American Herbalists Guild, PO Box 1127, Forestville, California 95436. Telephone 408 464 2441.

Northeast Herbal Association PO Box 146, Marshfield, VT 05658 0146.

QIGONG

China Advocates, 1635 Irving Street, San Francisco, CA 94122. Tel 415 665 4505.

Qigong Academy, 8103 Marlborough Avenue, Cleveland OH 44129. Telephone 216 842 9628.

Qigong Human Life Research Foundation, PO Box 5327, Cleveland OH 44101. Telephone 415 788 2227.

The Qigong Institute, East West Academy of Healing Arts, 450 Sutter Street, Suite 916, San Francisco, CA 94108. Telephone 818 564 9751.

Qigong Resource Associates, 1755 Homet Road, Pasadena, California 94122. Telephone 818 564 9751.

FURTHER READING

ACUPUNCTURE

Firebrace, Peter and Hill, Sandra *A Guide to Acupuncture* Constable.

Kenyon, Dr Julian *Modern techniques of Acupuncture* Thorsons.

Marcus, Dr Paul *Thorsons Introductory Guide to Acupuncture* Thorsons

Mole, Peter *Acupuncture, Energy Balancing for Body, Mind and Spirit* Element Books.

HERBS

Foster, Stephen and Chongxi, Yue *Herbal Emissaries* Healing Arts Press.

Tang, Stephen and Craze, Richard *Chinese Herbal Medicine* Piatkus.

QIGONG

Chuen, Master Lam Kan *The Way of Energy* Gaia Books Ltd.

Hongxun, Dr Shen *Taijiwuxigong* International Taijiwuxigong Institute.

Kiew Kit, Wong *The Art of Qigong* Element.

MacRitchie, James *Chi Kung* Element.

Quinn, Dr Khaleghl *Chi Kung* Thorsons.

Chengnan, Sun and Qilang, Wang *Chinese Massage Therapy* Shandong Science and Technology Press.

Li, Fan Ya *Chinese Pediatric Massage Therapy* Blue Poppy Press.

DIET

Flaws, Bob *Arisal of the Clear* Blue Poppy Press.

Jingfeng, Cai *Eating Your Way to Health* Foreign Languages Press, Beijing.

Leggett, Daverick *Helping Ourselves* Meridian Press.

GENERAL

Beinfeld, Harriet and Korngold, Efren *Between Heaven and Earth* Ballantyne Books.

Chang, Stephen T., *The Complete System of Chinese Self Healing* Thorsons.

Chih-Ling Koo, Linda *Nourishment of Life* Commercial Press Ltd, Hong Kong.

Kaptchuk, Ted *The Web That Has No Weaver* Rider Books.

Kenyon, Dr Julian *Acupressure for Health* Thorsons.

Mills, Simon *The Complete Guide to Modern Herbalism* Thorsons.

Page, Michael *The Power of Ch'i* Thorsons.

Quinn, Dr Khaleghl *Reclaim Your Power: The Secret Art of Maximising Your Potential* Thorsons.

Soo, Chee *The Chinese Art of Tai Chi Ch'uan* Thorsons.

Soo, Chee *The Tao of Long Life* Thorsons.

Thurman, Robert (trans) *Tibetan Secrets of Youth and Vitality* Thorsons.

Unschuld, Paul U., *Medicine in China. A History of Ideas* University of California Press.

Walters, Derek *Chinese Mythology* Thorsons.

Young, Jacqueline *Acupressure Techniques* Thorsons.

ANGELA HICKS

Angela Hicks qualified as an acupuncturist in 1976. She is Joint Principal of the College of Integrated Chinese Medicine in Reading, Berkshire, England. Besides teaching students she co-runs many post-graduate acupuncture courses. She regularly lectures in the US as well as practising and lecturing in England. She also practises qigong.

INDEX

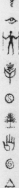

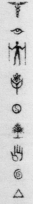